MW01675255

CASE MANAGEMENT ADHERENCE GUIDE 2020

CASE MANAGEMENT ADHERENCE GUIDE 2020

Case Management Society of America

cognella®
SAN DIEGO

Bassim Hamadeh, CEO and Publisher
Amy Smith, Senior Project Editor
Casey Hands, Production Editor
Jess Estrella, Senior Graphic Designer
Michaleigh Moylan, Licensing Associate
Natalie Piccotti, Director of Marketing
Kassie Graves, Vice President of Editorial
Jamie Giganti, Director of Academic Publishing

Primary author:
Rebecca Perez, MSN RN CCM
Case Management Society of America

Contributors:
Susan Rogers, MSN RN-BC CCM
Melanie Prince, MSN RN NEA-BC CCM FAAN
Kathleen Fraser, MSN MHA RN-BC FAAN CRRN CCM

Printed in the United States of America.

cognella® ACADEMIC PUBLISHING
3970 Sorrento Valley Blvd., Ste. 500, San Diego, CA 92121

This latest iteration of CMSA's *Case Management Adherence Guide* is dedicated to the CMSA leaders who had the vision and foresight to develop a resource for case managers that provides a patient-centered approach to support adherence and self-management resulting in improved health. *CMAG 2020* is built upon this strong foundation with up-to-date tools and strategies for today's changing health care landscape. This guide is specifically dedicated to CMSA past presidents Sherry Aliotta (2004–2005) and Susan Rogers (2005–2006). Always remember, *they* are the reason CMSA continues to bring you adherence guidance.

For more information about CMSA,
please visit www.cmsa.org.

BRIEF CONTENTS

DETAILED CONTENTS

FOREWORD

Why in the world would you read this? I am sure you are doing a job that is consuming all your energy, time, and brainpower. Our jobs are very challenging. But what do you do to show your worth? What is the outcome of your intervention with the client/patient? What should you do when the client is non-adherent? Why do you work so hard and have nothing to show for it as you have not met your goals for yourself, the client, or the full treatment team?

You should read or at least skim through this guide to find tools so you can achieve good outcomes with your interventions, making you more valuable to your employer, your client, and the treatment team. You will then know you are using appropriate tools and interventions. You are valuable! Show it!

In 2003, I was on the board of directors for national CMSA when I heard Sherry Aliotta, for the first time, describe outcomes of case management. Proving my case managers' worth was one thing I had been tasked to figure out for my employer. Managers in our system were financial people and wanted us to prove our worth financially. To prove our worth, we used scenarios such as "This is the amount of money saved based on the absence of surgeries," or "The patient was released 4 weeks before guidelines," or "The hospitalization was held to two days." Sherry was working with David Day, Pfizer's director of clinical applications, who educated other pharmacists and health care team members. They decided medication adherence was going to be huge in the pharmaceutical world and case managers would be ideal partners to help pharmacists and other treatment team members move their patients through the process of change management. Case Management Adherence Guidelines, along with a nationwide educational tour, were born.

By being on the national board, I had the opportunity to work with Sherry and a multitude of the brightest case managers. The collaboration was a true blessing. They were heroes to our organization and health care in general. This was one of the reasons I ran for the office of president.

I served as president of CMSA in 2005–2006 right behind Sherry, which gave me opportunities to further the idea of tools for the case manager. She is truly a champion of our organization and case managers.

CMAG soon became a guide and a piece of CMSA's Career and Knowledge Pathways. This puzzle piece fit right into the purpose of serving to drive best practice accountability for individual professional case managers and organizations. We designed our tools to "enhance understanding by expanding on these common principles to deliver a more unified education to professional case managers creating quality skill sets across the health care continuum" (CMSA). CMAG embraces the case management care continuum in any work environment, which contributes to consistency in foundational case management knowledge and a long, sustainable workforce. CMAG's evidence-based assessment tools provide case management professionals with evidence-based assessment and intervention tools to improve patient medication and treatment adherence.

So, back to the first question: Why should you read this or even skim to the addendum with the tools? We educate, empower our clients, coordinate care, and promote adherence.

Adherence is the cornerstone. If the client does not adhere to the treatment plan, the medication may not be effective, no empowerment takes hold, coordination of care does not matter because the client does not attend, and finally, it is a struggle for you to advocate.

I pride myself on being a case manager. I love the Case Management Society of America for giving me what I need for my practice and profession. I appreciate the case managers stepping up to continue the growth of the evidence-based and current practice tools. I love that 17 years ago, a fire began to burn around outcomes and CMSA fanned the flames for case management. I am very humbled by the opportunity to write the foreword to this new document.

Susan Rogers, MSN, RN-BC, CCM
CMSA President, 2005–2006

1

Challenges in Today's Health Care System

Kathleen Fraser, MSN, MHA, RN-BC, CCM, CRRN, FAAN

> *I have an almost complete disregard of precedent, and a faith in the possibility of something better. It irritates me to be told how things have always been done. I defy the tyranny of precedent. I go for anything new that might improve the past.*
>
> —Clara Barton

The health care field has undergone major changes, and health care workers must know how to integrate those new regulations, describe alternative payment options, and implement requirements for greater patient and family assessment, care planning, and care coordination into their practice. Individuals with complex medical conditions are typically a small percentage of the population but are responsible for using the greatest amount of our health care resources. An estimated 5% of the population uses 50% of health care resources, and those with five or more chronic conditions spend five times more for health care than those with no chronic conditions. This 5% of the population are those with comorbid medical and behavioral conditions. Fragmentation in care and lack of awareness of the need to link medical and mental conditions have resulted in higher health care costs and lack of quality of care received, leaving the infrastructure and tools not readily available to provide comprehensive services.

The Affordable Care Act has put a focus on the improvement of health outcomes, specifically calling out effective care coordination as activities to achieve these outcomes. Through collaboration, we can reduce duplications in health care, avoid gaps, and reduce health care costs. It involves continual communication with patients, their caregivers, and the various professionals and services with which they come into contact. The cumulative impact of multiple strategies (rather than single interventions) is more likely to be successful in improving patient experiences and outcomes and should be one of the key tools as part of a wider strategy. Evidence-based treatment is available for nearly every disease or condition, but implementation is inconsistent with strategies and tactics needed to address growth of medical and pharmaceutical costs and impacts to access and quality of care. Understanding, addressing, and assuring that all consumer interactions and outcomes are easy, convenient, timely, streamlined, and cohesive so health fits naturally into the "life flow" of the daily activities of every individual, family, and community remains the largest challenge.

According to the Agency for Health Care Research and Quality (AHRQ), the main goal of care coordination is to meet patients' needs and preferences in the delivery of high-quality, high-value health care. Care coordination is not a synonym for transition planning but a process that "ensures that the patients' health care needs and preferences are known and communicated at the right time, to the right people, and that this information is used to guide the delivery of safe, appropriate and effective care" (AHRQ, 2014). No one has had to weather more change than case managers due to the constant change in the regulatory environment, resulting in much scrutiny of the case manager role. Escalating costs, shifting payment methodologies, and increasingly complex populations are spawning new trends in care and reimbursement (for that care). A move outside of the acute care hospital to less costly settings and the community is underway. Health care spending in the United States totaled $3.5 trillion in 2017, with roughly 32% of that amount, or $1.1 trillion, spent on hospital services alone. Current hospital costs average approximately $3,949 per day, with each hospital stay averaging $15,734 (Fay, 2019). Avoidable health care expenses in the United States are estimated at $3.2 trillion, with continued growth estimated to be 5.5% by the year 2025 (Beaton, 2017).

Both the Centers for Medicare and Medicaid Services (CMS) and the payer community have emphasized a needed shift from volume to value. Hospitals and health care systems are scrambling to meet the expectations those new challenges demand (Fay, 2019). The development of value-based payment (VBP) programs, from Accountable Care Organizations (ACOs) to Bundle Payments for Care Improvement (BPCI) and Quality Payment Programs (QPPs), have forever altered how health care is rendered. Value will bring new attention to population health initiatives, and practitioners will shift focus to community-based care and wellness. The change will mandate the expertise of competent, credentialed case managers who meet defined qualifications and who acknowledge that care coordination extends beyond the walls of a single setting.

Dealing With This Challenge

Fundamental to the collaboration is the presence of the case manager, taking the responsibility for overseeing and coordinating that care and helping patients and caregivers navigate the system. The navigational role is important because most individuals selected for case management need services or input from one or more providers. By moving the case manager's focus away from tasks and procedures as the focus of their scope of practice, opportunities will be created to meet the needs of the health care consumer and add to the value of case managers (Lucatorto, 2016). Health care organizations must be purposeful in how they develop care teams and community partnerships that address the diverse needs of their populations. With most of the largest insurance companies developing programming to attend to the costliest populations (e.g., chronic care, integrated care, social determinants), seamless collaborative partnerships can be built among case managers across practice settings. Bridging the gap between volume and value is dependent on having a competent professional case management workforce that can coordinate care across the continuum and collaborate with care coordination colleagues from other provider or payer entities who are now attempting to see the hospitalized patients who are within their risk pools.

Many organizations collect outcomes and don't share the information, but case managers are there to communicate with all of the stakeholders to keep all of them on the same page to buy in to the process. Soft outcomes should not be overlooked, either. Patient, family, and provider satisfaction; the education of patients, family, and staff; advocating for patients and families to have the opportunity to assert their wishes; and assisting health care providers in communicating with patients effectively are all examples of soft outcomes that bring about the full transition of care without patients falling through the cracks. Operationalizing and scaling coordination and delivery system transformation of medical and non-medical services via partnerships and collaborations between health care and community-based organizations can overcome barriers, including social determinants of health, to effect better outcomes. Integrating and improving the exchange of member, payer, patient, and provider data and workflows can bring the value of aggregated data and systems on a near real-time and cost-effective basis to all stakeholders equitably. Identifying, addressing, and improving the member/patient's overall medical, lifestyle/behavioral, socioeconomic, cultural, financial, educational, geographic, and environmental well-being increases the chances for a frictionless and connected health care experience.

Turning Challenges Into Opportunities

Economically, the entire health care community is in turmoil, with one foot in the fee-for-service market while the other adjusts to various value-based payment and care delivery models that discourage inpatient admissions in favor of community-based care. As the marketplace undergoes these transformations, so must the vision of all case management programs. The greatest opportunity to drive down health costs—for payers, consumers, and the system in general—is with the payer-consumer relationship. A culture of engagement and accountability is essential for health systems to succeed in an era of population health management and accountable care. Strong organizational cultures enable and nurture the new behaviors, actions, and investments required to navigate the many changes affecting the health care industry, particularly the transition to value-based care. But driving cultural improvement is not easy, and it does not happen overnight. To the contrary, efforts to change culture must consider the history, heritage, and attitudes of an organization's past. And they must be carefully and continually assessed, developed, and nurtured at all levels of the organization, developing and integrating technical and operational infrastructure and programs for a more collaborative and equitable approach to manage costs, share risk, and enhance quality outcomes in the transition from volume to value.

With multiple stakeholders trying to manage a patient's care, there is immense opportunity for enhanced stakeholder interoperability to reduce disparate systems of care and align a network on one centralized platform. Providers should use care coordination across the continuum in a way that is meaningful and actionable. According to Kaiser Family Foundation research, the annual cost of a family health insurance plan has now surpassed $20,000. Some of the primary reasons include escalating drug prices (particularly for specialty drugs), high-cost therapies coming to market, and industry consolidation. Payers and providers should continue their efforts to be a part of the solution, working to partner to help solve the problems that contribute to the high cost of health care. In addition, they should increase their focus on innovative solutions to the problem—what can be done differently to enhance efficiency and effectiveness, both in terms of improving what is working and fixing what's not. Diligently monitoring and understanding these changes is critical, as is making sure they are aligned with the best industry solutions in the space. Also consider their effect on programs such as value-based care and established clinical pathways.

U.S. health care—especially its cost and delivery—will be top of mind in 2020 and beyond. A new value-based marketplace calls for a new vision of case management that eschews tasks and instead focuses on activities that promote a safe, coordinated journey across the continuum for the most vulnerable patients. DIY health care takes on new meaning as American consumers will begin to finally reap benefits from the enormous investments in data collection, storage, and analysis that have been made by the U.S. health industry. Beyond offering them tools to monitor their vitals, at-home devices to test for strep throat or flu, or personal health records that consumers themselves must populate, companies are building business models around giving consumers access to their own data with insights attached. New entrants are pulling together electronic health records, claims data, steps, lab work, sleep patterns, and more to give consumers a holistic view of their health and where it is heading. Case managers find themselves at the forefront of facilitating greater collaboration amongst providers who have been accustomed to substantial autonomy.

And lastly, if you are truly going to have a case management department that can carry out the value adds to their greatest potential and turn these health care challenges into opportunities, you must allow them to case manage. True care coordination can only occur through the essential interaction with patients, families, and other health care team members. If not, you are doing utilization management, not case management, and the opportunities are lost and only the challenges remain!

References

Agency for Health Care Research and Quality (AHRQ). (2014). What is care coordination? *Care Coordination Measures Atlas Update*. https://www.ahrq.gov/ncepcr/care/coordination/atlas/chapter2.html

Appold, K. (2020). Top 6 challenges healthcare executives will face in 2020. *Managed Healthcare Executive.* https://www.managedhealthcareexecutive.com/view/top-6-challenges-healthcare-executives-will-face-2020

Beaton, T. (2017). Top 10 most expensive chronic diseases for health care payers. HealthPayerIntelligence. https://healthpayerintelligence.com/news/top-10-most-expensive-chronic-diseases-for-healthcare-payers

Case Management Society of America. (2020). What is a Case Manager? https://cmsa.org/who-we-are/what-is-a-case-manager/#:~:text=Case%20Management%20is%20a%20collaborative,quality%20of%20care%2C%20and%20cost

Fay, B. (2019). Hospital and surgery costs. Debt.org. https://www.debt.org/medical/hospital-surgery-costs/

Fraser, K., Perez, R., & Latour, C. (Eds.). (2018). *CMSA's integrated case management: A manual for case managers by case managers.* Springer Publishing Company.

Gooch, K. (2018, October 25) Social determinants of health contributes to over half of readmissions. *Becker's Hospital Review.* https://www.beckershospitalreview.com/care-coordination/social-determinants-of-health-contributed-to-half-of-hospital-readmissions-study-finds.html

Henry J. Kaiser Family Foundation. (2020). Kaiser Family Foundation Poll: February 2020 Kaiser Health Tracking Poll (Version 3) [Dataset]. Cornell University, Ithaca, NY: Roper Center for Public Opinion Research. doi:10.25940/ROPER-31117209

Lucatorto, M. A., Thomas, T. W., Siek, T. (September 30, 2016). Registered nurses as caregivers: Influencing the system as patient advocates. *OJIN: The Online Journal of Issues in Nursing, 21*(3[2]). http://ojin.nursingworld.org/MainMenuCategories/ANAMarketplace/ANAPeriodicals/OJIN/TableofContents/Vol-21-2016/No3-Sept-2016/Registered-Nurses-as-Caregivers-Influencing-the-System-as-PatientAdvocates.html

Why we need public health to improve healthcare. National Association of Chronic Disease Directors. https://www.chronicdisease.org/page/whyweneedph2imphc.

Young, K., Hunzinger, G., Singh, G., & Isgur, B. (2021). Top health industry issues of 2021: Will a shocked system emerge stronger? *PwC.* https://www.pwc.com/us/en/industries/health-industries/top-health-industry-issues.html

2

The Important Role Case Managers Play in Improving Outcomes

Melanie Prince, MSS, MSN, RN, NEA-BC, FAAN

Case managers fulfill many roles in health care settings, and case managers' dexterity and chameleon-like ability to make adaptive role changes is a hallmark trait. Case managers' inherent, learned, and experiential leadership skills are critically important to honing in on the factors leading to improved health outcomes, especially with patient adherence.

Leadership behaviors in the clinical setting mirror the same leadership styles as those in other professional settings. An Internet literature search confirms five to seven types of leadership styles: autocratic, authoritarian, pacesetting, democratic, coaching, affiliative, and laissez-faire. Any of these styles can exert influence on a patient's behavior, but case managers must complement these leadership techniques by taking on another role: investigator.

The case manager investigator must first evaluate their personal attitudes toward the patient's situation in totality. It is important to reflect on possible inherent bias, judgments related to social-cultural circumstances or personal barriers that may hinder one from becoming a full partner in the journey toward consistent adherence. This "reflective investigation" into oneself is the first step to identifying the best leadership style to employ when motivating patients for adherence and improved outcomes. The second step is to investigate the patient's worldview of their health situation.

A patient's worldview of health management is framed within social and physical determinants of health, as described in Table 2.1.

TABLE 2.1

Social Determinants	Physical Determinants
- Availability of resources to meet daily needs (e.g., safe housing and local food markets) - Access to educational, economic, and job opportunities - Access to health care services - Quality of education and job training - Availability of community-based resources in support of community living and opportunities for recreational and leisure-time activities - Transportation options - Public safety - Social support - Social norms and attitudes (e.g., discrimination, racism, and distrust of government) - Exposure to crime, violence, and social disorder (e.g., presence of trash and lack of cooperation in a community) - Socioeconomic conditions (e.g., concentrated poverty and the stressful conditions that accompany it) - Residential segregation - Language/literacy - Access to mass media and emerging technologies (e.g., cell phones, the Internet, and social media) - Culture	- Natural environment, such as green space (e.g., trees and grass) or weather (e.g., climate change) - Built environment, such as buildings, sidewalks, bike lanes, and roads - Worksites, schools, and recreational settings - Housing and community design - Exposure to toxic substances and other physical hazards - Physical barriers, especially for people with disabilities - Aesthetic elements (e.g., good lighting, trees, and benches)

Source: Office of Disease Prevention and Health Promotion. Social determinants of health. Healthy People 2020. *https://www.healthypeople.gov/2020/topics-objectives/topic/social-determinants-of-health*

In addition to these determinants, the case manager, as investigator, must also assess the patient's sense of value. Value-based care is not solely from the institutional perspective but also, importantly, from the patient perspective. It is the patient who determines what aspect of health management is most important to them. This value determinant may range from wanting to live to reducing physical symptoms or avoiding aesthetic symptoms. David Ebbevi and associates conducted a study, "Value-Based Health Care for Chronic Care: Aligning Outcomes Measurement With the Patient Perspective." While the study is limited to a specific disease state, the premise that discovering patients' preferred outcomes is interesting in that it reflects directly on one's willingness to engage in consistent behaviors of adherence to a treatment plan.

The case manager, in an investigatory role, should validate the patient's preferred outcomes, examine the social and physical determinants with which the patient (and influencers) exist, and apply the leadership style that will encourage engagement and partnership. Whether transactional or pacesetting, coaching or taking an affiliative approach, case managers have the skills to influence a variety of situations and settings that drive adherence and achieve mutually determined health outcomes.

Reference

Ebbevi, D., et al. (2016). Value-based health care for chronic care: Aligning outcomes measurement with the patient perspective. *Quality Management in Health Care* 25(4): 203–212.

3

Adherence

Chronic diseases are now common in the United States, with about 117 million people having at least one chronic illness, at a cost of $1.3 trillion in direct health care costs and lost productivity (Abbass, 2017). The World Health Organization published its most recent statistics in 2018, and the United States per capita health care expenditures are $9,403 (World Health Organization, 2018). These expenditures are 17.1% of our gross national product, or GDP (WHO, 2018). The average life expectancy for males in the United States is 76 years, and 86 years for females (WHO, 2018). Life expectancy has increased in the United States, but as people are living longer, they are doing so with chronic illness. Chronic diseases are the major cause of death and disability worldwide (WHO, 2018). In the United States, chronic disease accounts for 88% of all deaths, and the major contributor to chronic disease is a raised BMI (obesity and overweight), with the trend expected to continue (WHO, 2018).

Medication nonadherence is a public health concern resulting from the growth in the numbers of Americans with chronic illnesses (Abbass, 2017). The context of nonadherence includes the presence of multiple chronic conditions, cost, and psychological, social, and health system challenges. Fifty percent of Americans do not adhere to their prescribed medications causing adverse health outcomes, ED utilization, increased costs in care, and reduced workforce productivity (Abbass, 2017). Medication nonadherence can have a greater impact on patient outcomes than the specific treatment itself (NACDS, 2017). Nonadherence accounts for 50% of treatment failures and up to 25% of hospitalizations (NACDS, 2017).

The Business Case for Adherence

The cost of nonadherence is significant, causing 125,000 deaths and $100–$289 billion per year (NACDS, 2017). Treatment failures result in medical resource utilization, and new problems develop as a result of nonoptimized medication use (August, 2018). The National Association of Chain Drug Stores reported the following in 2017 (NACDS, 2017):

- Nonadherence increases the risk of dying tenfold over homicide
- 89,000 deaths occur as a result of hypertension medication nonadherence behaviors
    - One in two individuals miss doses
    - One in three forget if they have taken their medication
    - One in four do not refill the prescription on time
- One in five Medicare patients is readmitted within 30 days, with 50% of those admissions related to medication nonadherence
- 41%–59% of mental health patients do not take medications as prescribed, if at all
- 50% of people with a chronic condition stop taking medications within one year
- 20%–30% of all prescriptions are never filled
- 50% of prescribed medications for chronic conditions are not taken as directed

Most people do not make conscious decisions to stop taking medication. The most common causes of nonadherence are as follows (NACDS, 2017):

- Inattention/procrastination (69%)
- Cost (16%)
- Side effects or lack of response (15%)

Most often, people forget to take their medications, get out of the habit of taking them, and then stop taking them altogether. Adherence to prescribed treatment, including medications, contributes to positive health outcomes and reduces the need for costly interventions, such as hospital admissions (Tueller & Deboeck, 2016). Research tells us that a 10% improvement in medication adherence reduces up to 29% of costs, and for every 1% improvement in adherence, $50 is saved in health care spending (NACDS, 2017). One employment study showed that adherence improved productivity by $18,000 per employee per year (NACDS, 2017).

The evidence that adherence reduces costs is strong enough to impact policy. Medicare Advantage plans offer incentives to physicians who meet quality and pay-for-performance measures. Accountable Care Organizations are also incentivized to implement best practices related to pharmacy collaboration and patient education about medication self-management. The challenge with adherence is helping patients adopt and maintain behaviors that promote wellness, prevent illness, and encourage self-management (Volpp, 2018).

Why Is Adherence Easy for Some and Hard for Others?

Individuals do not decide one day to just stop taking insulin and checking blood sugar as a treatment for diabetes—people are generally not that obstinate or stubborn. Instead, there are many factors that lead to a lack of adherence. What needs to happen is a discovery of what is interfering in an individual's ability to self-manage and then address the interferences.

Adherence varies across individuals and is generally a trade-off between short-term effort and long-term benefit. An individual's attitude about risk plays a role in adherence: those who are risk-averse have higher rates of adherence, while those who can be considered risk-seeking have lower rates of adherence. There is a need to acknowledge and accommodate innovations to promote self-management. Evidence suggests that leveraging the potential of every individual to care for themselves and involving them in decisions that affect their health is beneficial (Dineen-Griffin, Garcia-Cardenas, & Williams, 2019).

The "secret sauce" to support self-management is a combination of the use of evidence with a patient-centered approach. When patients participate in their health care decisions, the gap between patient and provider narrows. But to accomplish this, patients must be engaged with their providers, exchange knowledge, set goals, and carry out self-management activities. Patients and providers become partners, and this partnership results in better symptom control, especially for those with chronic conditions (Dineen-Griffin, Garcia-Cardenas, & Williams, 2019). Self-management is essential to chronic disease management and prevention but must be tailored to the individual's preferences and circumstances. Self-management requires a cache of tools and techniques that help the individual choose healthy behaviors and a fundamental change in the patient–provider relationship to one of a collaborative partnership.

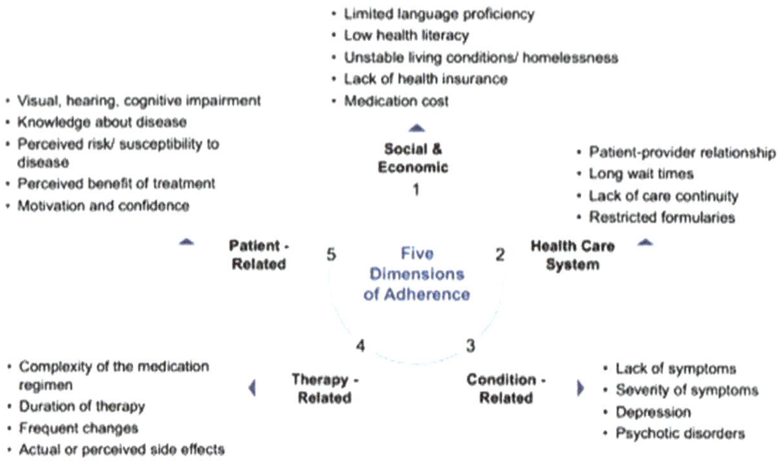

FIGURE 3.1 Diagram Outlining the Factors Related to Nonadherence.

The challenges of adherence have not changed much over the years, so moving patients to self-management remains a work in progress. There are multiple reasons nonadherence occurs, but the most often reported are forgetfulness, concerns about cost, and side effects. Adherence encompasses a mutual agreement to adhere to therapeutic components following a professional diagnosis and evidence-based treatment recommendations with the overarching goal of attaining the best possible outcomes in the long term (Montague, 2017).

In addition to forgetfulness, contributors to nonadherence include lack of knowledge and understanding of the rationale for treatment as well as social and psychological challenges. More than one-half of individuals believe that education about preventable conditions is effective at initiating behavior change, but only one-fourth believe this intervention is sustaining behavior change (Volpp, 2018). There are three interventions that are preferred by patients:

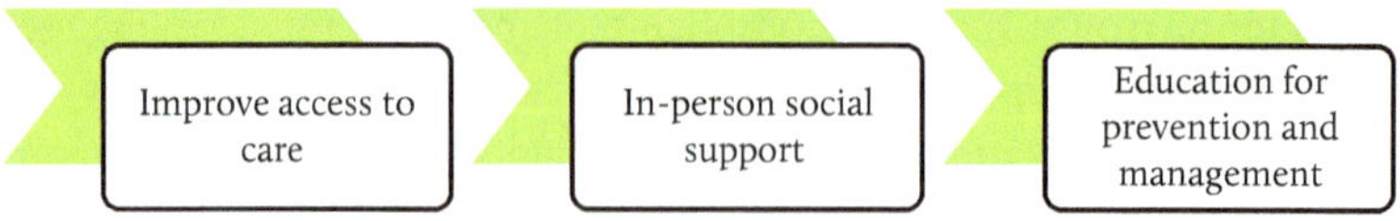

FIGURE 3.2 Three Interventions.

Only one intervention has been noted by patients to be the most helpful in initiating and sustaining behavior change, and that is in-person social support (Volpp, 2018). Sixty-three percent of patients say that in-person support helped them initiate behavior change, and 64% said in-person support sustained their behavior change (Volpp, 2018).

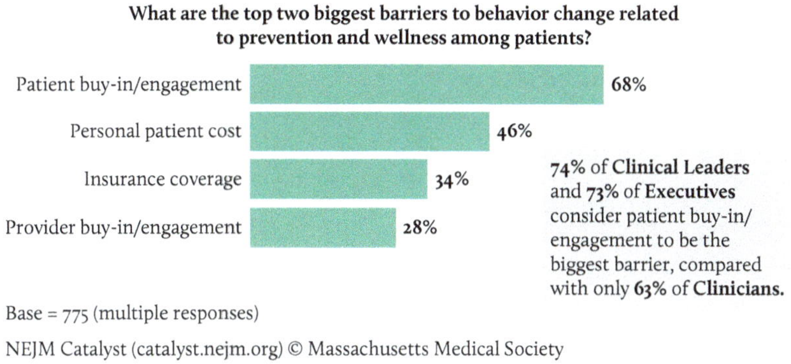

FIGURE 3.3 Patient Engagement Is the Biggest Barrier to Behavior Change.

Physicians often encourage behavior change by providing advice on consequences (van der Pol, 2017). Providers often do not have the time to initiate and sustain behavior change because they must focus on treating disease and acting quickly to address acute issues. Many approaches found to be effective in the management of chronic disease are not under the direct control of providers. For example, the physician cannot write a prescription for a family to become more involved in a patient's care or order friends to visit. When providers prescribe interventions to support adherence that are not covered by insurance plans, the provider is seen as the "bad guy" because the patient now has an additional financial burden related to the treatment of their condition. Interestingly, providers agree with patients as to the most effective means of initiating and sustaining behavior change: education, social support, and financial incentives (Volpp, 2018). The least effective are personal devices like FitBit, wellness applications, and financial penalties (Volpp, 2018).

Conclusion

In this chapter, the relationship of chronic illness and nonadherence has been clearly defined along with the cyclical impact of one on the other. This introduction to adherence will be followed with more detail about the challenges of adherence and recommendations to improve it, including tools and demonstrations by other organizations. Specific areas of concentration will be care coordination and transition of care, as these are integral to supporting clients/patients in adherence and better health outcomes.

Putting It Into Practice

Ask yourself these questions to target interventions for improvement

- What are the causes of poorly controlled chronic conditions?
- Is poor adherence one of those causes?
- Have admissions to the hospital or ED resulted from poor adherence?
- If your client/patient were adherent, what health improvements would you expect?
- Would those improvements equate to reduced health care spending?
- Have you included in your assessments the true causes of nonadherence (do not assume the individual is difficult, obstinate, or stubborn)?
- How can you better engage your client/patient?
- Do they have what they need to access care?
- Do they have a relationship with a provider?
- Who is available to provide support?

References

Abbass, I. R. (2017). Medication nonadherence: The role of cost, community, and individual factors. *Health Research and Educational Trust, 52*(4), 1511–1533.

August, T. (2018). Cost of inappropriate use of medication. *Pharmacy Times.*

Boylan, L. (2017). *The cost of medication nonadherence.* Alexandria, VA: National Association of Chain Drug Stores.

Dineen-Griffin, S., Garcia-Cardenas, V., & Williams, K. (2019). Helping patients help themselves: A systematic review of self-management support strategies in primary health care practice. *PLOS ONE, 14*(8). doi:https://doi.org/10.1371/journal.pone.0220116

Montague, T., Manness, L., Cochrane, B., Gogovor, A., Aylen, J., Martin, L., & Nemis-white, J. (2017). Non-adherence to prescribed therapy: A persistent contributor to the care gap. *HCIC*, 1–9.

Tueller, S., & Deboeck, P. (2016). Getting less of what you want: Reductions in statistical power and increased bias when categorizing adherence data. *Journal of Behavioral Health, 39*, 969–980. doi:10.1007/s10865-016-9727-9

van der Pol, M. H. (2017). The role of time and risk preferences in adherence to physician advice on health behavior change. *European Journal of Health Economics, 18*, 373–386. doi:10.1007/s10198-016-0800-7

Volpp, K. G. (2018). *What creates behavior change may not sustain it.* Waltham, MA: NEJM Catalyst.

World Health Organization. (2018). *World health statistics.* Geneva, Switzerland: World Health Organization.

Figure Credits

Fig. 3.1: Adapted from Eduardo Sabaté, "Diagram Outlining the Factors Related to Non-Adherence," Adherence to Long-term Therapies: Evidence for Action. Copyright © 2003 by Massachusetts Medical Society.

Fig. 3.3: Source: https://catalyst.nejm.org/doi/full/10.1056/CAT.18.0173.

4

Improving Adherence

Engagement and Retention

Adherence to medication or other prescribed treatment is not as simple as one would think. Reasons for nonadherence range from forgetfulness to avoidance due to condition-related stigma. Adherence does not necessarily result from a provider instructing a patient on what medications to take but comes more from the patient understanding why they are taking medication. Adherence will happen if the patient is engaged in their health care.

Some researchers consider a patient engaged if they participate in studies or use study tools (Sieck, Walker, & Retchin, 2019). Scales have been developed that measure psychological and emotional states that indicate engagement (Sieck, Walker, & Retchin, 2019). Others examine behaviors such as preparing for a medical appointment in advance or making medication lists as measures of adherence (Sieck, Walker, & Retchin, 2019). These measures fall short because they do not measure the context in which a patient engages: whether the patient has a trusted relationship with a provider, is able to get convenient appointments, and has adequate financial resources to access needed care (Sieck, Walker, & Retchin, 2019).

Sieck et al., from the Center for the Advancement of Team Science, Analytics, and Systems Thinking in Health Services and Implementation Science Research (CATALYST) at Ohio State University, developed the Engagement Capacity Framework (Figure 4.1). The framework encompasses four dimensions that fall within the domains of person,

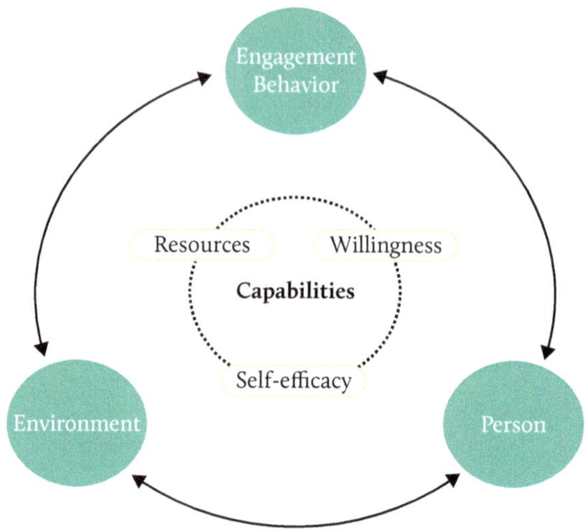

FIGURE 4.1 Engagement Capacity Framework.

environment, and behavior (Sieck, Walker, & Retchin, 2019). Sieck et al. included the theory of reciprocal determinism in their model because of the dynamic relationships among the person, the environment, and their behaviors. These continually influence and are influenced by each other. For example, when an individual learns a new behavior, such as cooking low-fat foods that really taste good, as time goes by, the individual's confidence grows, and the behavior continues (Sieck, Walker, & Retchin, 2019).

The following is detailed information about the Engagement Capacity Framework (ECF) Dimensions (Sieck, Walker, & Retchin, 2019):

Defining the ECF Dimensions

Understanding an individual's capacity for engagement means identifying and understanding the elements and dimensions that influence the domains.

Self-efficacy is the individual's belief in their own capability to perform or adopt a behavior. Increases in self-efficacy have been linked to chronic disease management, adherence to treatment plans, and healthier behaviors.

Resources are external factors that support an individual in their care, such as income and health insurance, Internet access and patient portals or other patient-specific materials, availability of convenient appointments, and a trusted patient–provider relationship.

(Continued)

Defining the ECF Dimensions (Continued)

Willingness is being ready to act. Many providers are accessible online, but if the patient is distrustful of this means of communication, engagement is hindered.

Capabilities are the knowledge and skills that enable an individual to perform a behavior. This can mean knowing where and what information to access.

It is important to understand these dimensions from the patient's perspective. Here are some examples:

Self-efficacy: access to blood work results before an appointment so the results can be discussed. Instead of the patient having to write down questions for the next appointment, a patient portal allows for questions to be answered in real time, the ability to make and track appointments, and the capability to track test results.

Resources: spouses included in support group discussions or education classes to reinforce the information received; access to a patient portal with educational resources.

Willingness: questioning the physician when something is not understood or sharing what has or has not worked in the past rather than passively listening to the physician.

Capabilities: repeating back instructions given; asking for written instructions in addition to verbal instructions in case questions arise; being more assertive to make sure your voice is heard.

Capacity and context help clinicians better understand the needs of the individual as well as a population. Consider the following:

1. Patient is newly diagnosed with diabetes but is unable to access testing supplies—**Low Resources**
2. A patient newly diagnosed with diabetes lacks the confidence to self-inject insulin—**Low Self-Efficacy**
3. A patient newly diagnosed with insulin-dependent diabetes has a fear of needles—**Low Willingness**

Each of these situations requires a different intervention. The low-resources individual needs financial assistance to gain access to supplies, whether that means enrollment in a scholarship program, discounted supplies, or a brand of supplies that is less expensive. The low-self-efficacy patient needs support and coaching. This can be done in the outpatient setting or by a home health nurse to coach and encourage the ability to self-inject. The low-willingness patient requires more specialized interventions: perhaps a spouse or other family member can administer the insulin for a brief time or instruct on using devices that are less like needles, such as injection pens. Regardless of the approach, this situation will take time, patience, and support.

Patient engagement is seen as the missing piece necessary to improve direct care and patient experience (Angove & Boselovic, 2018). Clinicians are now focusing on patient-centered care to improve engagement. There is no universally accepted definition or set of principles for patient-centered care, but some nationally recognized institutions have offered definitions and principles and are being recognized for their approach to patient-centered care. With the *New England Journal of Medicine*'s list of seven principles of patient-centered care as inspiration, the Mountain States Health Alliance (MSHA) was recognized by the National Quality Forum and *Becker's Hospital Review* in 2012 for its 10 Principles for Patient-Centered Care (Angove & Boselovic, 2018; see Figure A.3, Appendix 14):

1. All team members are caregivers
2. Care is based on continuous healing relationships
3. Care is customized and reflects the patient's needs, preferences, and values
4. Knowledge and information are freely shared between and among patients, care partners, physicians, and other caregivers
5. Care is provided in a healing environment of comfort, peace, and support
6. Families and friends of the patient are considered
7. Patient safety is a visible priority
8. Transparency is the rule in the care of the patient
9. All caregivers cooperate with one another through a common focus on the best interests and personal goals of the patient
10. The patient is the source of control for their care

Listening to the Patient's Voice

Historically and, unfortunately, currently, health care systems design care around the needs and convenience of providers and institutions. Centering resources around infrastructure works well in many other industries, but not in health care. The design of any care or care structure should center around patients.

Patients should have a voice in the design of all aspects of health care, whether it be physical spaces or workflows. Establishing patient-family advisory committees is a good way to gather information about what matters to patients and families (Angove & Boselovic, 2018). Such committees support the codevelopment and coproduction of care and provider–patient activities that impact health outcomes (Angove & Boselovic, 2018).

Das, Abramson, and Kaushal share the "voice of the patient" with results from research sponsored by the Patient-Centered Outcomes Research Institute. Several focus groups were conducted with high-cost, high-needs patients to inquire about what things would improve their abilities to manage health conditions. They identified five solutions that would reduce utilization of the emergency department (ED) and hospital admissions (Tanmoy Das, Abramson, & Kaushal, 2019):

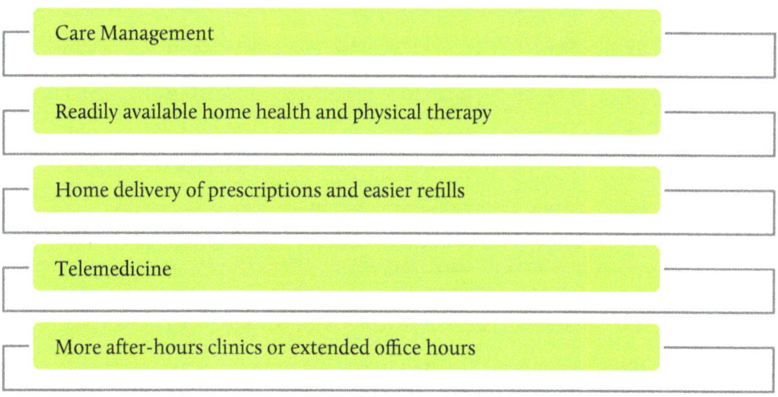

FIGURE 4.2 Five Solutions.

Health outcomes have moved from the collection of objective data to incorporation of the patient's voice into health data. Biometrics are also now being included in data for health outcomes, such as hours of sleep and number of steps per day, which can be predictors of risk and assist in targeting interventions, as are **patient-reported outcome measures** (**PROMs**; Wagle, 2019). Patient-reported outcome measures quantify a patient's symptoms, physical function, mood/mental health, and quality of life (QOL; Wagle, 2019). A suggested method for quantifying PROMs is the use of numerical scales that allow monitoring of improvement or decline and guides implementation of interventions specific to the reported issue (Wagle, 2019). Examples of PROMs can be found in Appendix 2. The following are patient comments published by clients/patients:

Solution	Quote
Care management	It's (care coordination) (that is) very useful. She gave me the thing to call her, and I could call her at any time I'm feeling bad. I tell you, most of it is anxiety. So, when I talk to her it calms me down, and she also helps me out, she said take some—over-the-counter medication that helps me that I don't have to run to the emergency room, and she'll tell me why not to go to the emergency room.
At-home services (visiting nurse/physical therapy)	Having a home nurse come to your home or a physical therapist come to your home. Because I had both of them come to my house when I had my hips replaced. Both of them because there wasn't no sense—because I didn't want to go from the hospital to a rehab hospital and stay in the hospital more. I had the ... the home nurse and then I had my home therapist come to the house. That stopped me from having to go to the hospital.
At-home medication delivery	You have to go every month and pick that prescription up. Sometimes that can be hard. Sometimes you can't make it there to get it and you do without it. I think they need to come up with a way where when they know it's time for you to come there to pick that prescription up, either mail that prescription home to them or something like that.
Larger supply of medications	They give you your medication—if instead of giving you a 30-day supply, they give you a 90-day supply and give it to you so that when you get to that last prescription bottle, you can go ahead and put that order in so that you can go ahead and get that next 90-day supply. That'll help a lot.
Telemedicine	I think that might help, 'Cause like he says, most of it comes with anxiety. If you could talk to somebody that knows your symptoms and feels comfortable talking, yeah, and explain to them what's going on, they could just let you know this is what's going on. You've been through it before, it's nothing. And also, it relaxes you. The whole idea of telemedicine works fine except that most practitioners. If they're at all concerned about it being cardiac, prefer that you get your behind over there so you can get looked at. Okay. And so, I mean, that's what I've been led to belive that there's no point in taking a chance because the price and consequences is much too great.
After-hours clinics	Instead of people ... going to the emergency room a lot—have y'all ever thought about like opening up a clinic like after hours after the regular clinic is closed? Have y'all ever thought about like opening that up to solve some of the problems that, you know, they won't have to go to the emergency room quite so frequently?

FIGURE 4.3 What High-Need, High-Cost Patients Say About How to Reduce High Utilization of ED and Inpatient Services.

Contributors to poor outcomes

-Health-related social needs, or social determinants of health, contribute more to poor health outcomes than any other health care barrier or concern (Sieck, Walker, & Retchin, 2019). If a patient has unsafe housing, not enough to eat, an inability to pay for medicines, or feels threatened in their community, focusing on health is not a priority.

-The type of health information provided can vary from individual to individual. Having access to channels and formats of communication that meet the patient's preference is crucial to the ability to fully comprehend health information. Communication in person or by text, phone call, email, or written correspondence are acceptable methods for most patients and families.

-Social isolation can be deadly. Whether living alone or without the support of family and friends, isolation is detrimental to care, especially if the patient has suffered a recent acute episode.

(Das, Abramson, & Kaushal, 2019)

Patient Experience

Patient experience not only refers to satisfaction with care received or improvements in quality of life but also includes peace of mind—the reassurance that everything that should be done is being done and going forward, the patient will receive what is needed; how a patient's care journey progresses contributes to satisfaction (Wagle, 2019). A patient whose expectations were met or exceeded will be satisfied with the care experience.

Patients today expect health care to be more in line with other consumer experiences, such as with an Internet provider or retailer. Access to non-health services is much easier than it once was, and patients now expect this with health care. The "instant gratification" consumers receive when purchasing items online has resulted in the demand for care and answers to be delivered quickly but also with a personal touch. Not surprisingly, more than 80% of health care consumers are dissatisfied with their health care experiences (Wagle, 2019). Health care has been slow to adopt a consumer-centric approach, but patients are making their preferences known, clearly indicating what would improve their health care experience. **The same on-demand services available in the world of business are desired in health care**. Patients want to be able to self-schedule appointments, communicate with their providers directly via text messages or emails, have access to video chats and virtual appointments, be able to pay their bills online, and receive reminders and other health information via texts and emails. These digital tools will improve engagement for more than 50% of the population (Wagle, 2019). Digital tools may be less popular or accessible for those who are less technology-savvy or those lacking online or digital resources.

Access to Care

It is no secret that the way to promote and maintain health, prevent and manage disease, reduce disability, and prevent premature death is by improving access to needed health services. The top three requirements for accessing care are insurance coverage or a way to pay for care, the physical availability of health services, and timeliness of care delivery (Office of Disease Prevention and Health Promotion, 2019). These are accomplished with (ODPHP, 2019):

- Entry into a health system
- Geographic availability of services
- Location of a provider who is trusted, communicates well, and is willing to develop a personal relationship

Barriers exist that prevent access to care and results in health inequities. These barriers include (ODPHP, 2019):

- The high cost of care
- Inadequate or no insurance coverage
- Lack of available services

Barriers to accessing care result in (ODPHP, 2019):

- Unmet health needs
- Delays in receiving care
- Inability to access preventative care
- Financial burdens
- Preventable hospitalizations

How and where care is accessed is influenced by (ODPHP, 2019):

- Age
- Race
- Ethnicity
- Socioeconomic status
- Sex
- Disability status
- Sexual orientation
- Gender identity
- Residential location

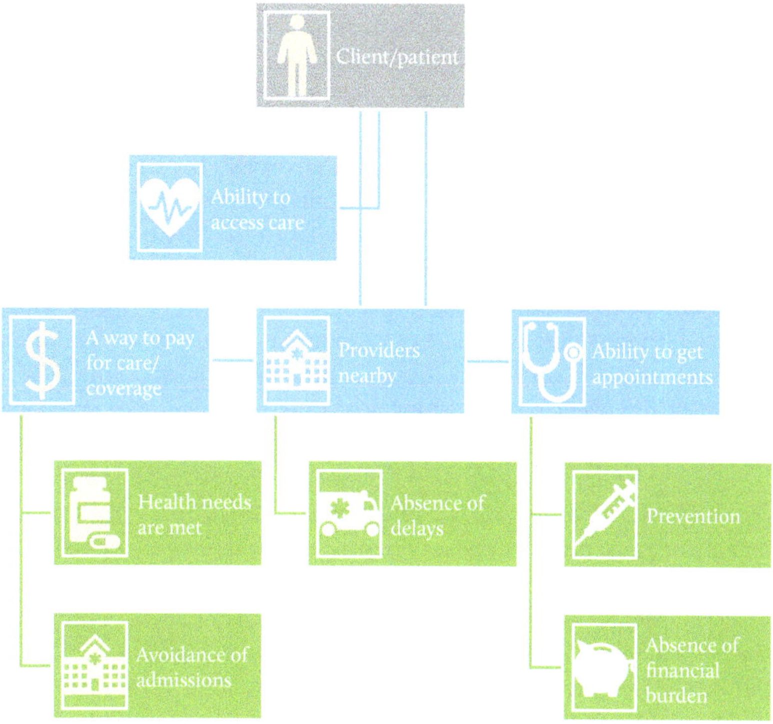

FIGURE 4.4 Requirements for Access to Care.

Having health insurance coverage allows entry into the health care system. Lack of or inadequate coverage makes it difficult or impossible to get care. If care is accessed without any health coverage, a financial burden is the result. Those who have inadequate or no health coverage are more likely to be sicker and less likely to access care, are diagnosed with conditions later in the sequalae, and are more likely to die prematurely (ODPHP, 2019).

Access to care can be improved if an individual is able to develop a trusted relationship with a primary care provider. Trust, shared decisions, and communication with a provider indicate the right care will be received at the right time, decreasing the risk of disability or premature death. Timeliness of care access is essential to prevent worsening conditions, admissions, emotional distress, and higher treatment costs. Delays in care negatively impact health and costs. These can be avoided by making appointments available when illness or injury occurs: for example, keeping appointment slots open for urgent situations or extending office hours into the evening. If appointments are not available when a client/patient needs one, ED use rises.

According to Healthy People 2020, 89.7% of Americans had health coverage in 2017, which was an increase from 83.1% in 2012 (ODPHP, 2019). But even with this increase, only 76.8% had primary care providers. In 2015, only 76.4% of covered Americans had primary care providers, so even with an increase in coverage, the rate of having primary care providers did not significantly increase (ODPHP, 2019). The goal, of course, would be for all Americans to have access to care, and while the number of individuals with coverage is encouraging, it is not all-inclusive. Equally of concern is the number of Americans with health coverage who do not have primary care providers. This means there are many Americans accessing care from specialists only, urgent care centers, or emergency departments and are not receiving preventative services.

Having health coverage does not automatically ensure improved access to care. For example, Medicaid enrollees are less likely to get timely appointments scheduled; those with private insurance will typically get appointments quicker (Hsiang, et al., 2019). Not every provider is willing to accept Medicaid patients. In a nationwide survey conducted in 2015, only 45% of providers were willing to accept new Medicaid patients, but 94% were open to accepting new patients with private insurance (Hsiang et al., 2019). This is attributed to Medicaid's low reimbursement levels, a disadvantaged population, and high administrative burden (Hsiang et al., 2019). These all contribute to the health disparities experienced by Medicaid enrollees. According to Hsiang et al., while Medicaid patients have more difficulty getting appointments, once they access care, appropriate care is received (Hsiang et al., 2019). Delays in care and difficulty developing trusted provider relationships are of concern. Even though Medicaid coverage was expanded with the Patient Protection and Affordable Care Act and more individuals were covered, obtaining appointments remains difficult.

Whether an individual is covered by Medicaid, Medicare, the Veterans Administration, federal programs such as TRICARE, faith-based insurers, Indian Health Services, or private insurance, other contributors to poor access are social determinants of health (SDOH). These include environment, culture, ethnicity, nutrition, education, and finances. If present, these determinants need to be addressed holistically—assessing the individual and not the condition, exploring what may be in the community to assist, understand cultural impact, and be responsive. Addressing SDOH is best accomplished when health care providers partner with organizations in a community to provide resources and services that will improve health (Spruce, 2019). Examples of utilizing community resources include (Spruce, 2019):

- Developing relationships with mental health providers who work with and advocate for victims of violence
- Knowing where food pantries are located, especially those that supply food for families at no charge
- Knowing where homeless people can access care
- Developing legal partnerships to help families and individuals with legal services
- Finding resources to assist those who are underinsured

Individuals often cannot control the SDOH that affect them and may not know how or where to get help (Spruce, 2019). Unhealthy behaviors are the result of a response to the current environment. Health care providers must know and understand these obstacles so strategies can be developed. For example, an individual struggling with obesity may not have access to healthy food or have a safe place to exercise. Addressing SDOH requires compassion and empathy. Questions need to be asked without judgment, and inquiries can be phrased in a way that helps identify problems and challenges. When a nonthreatening,

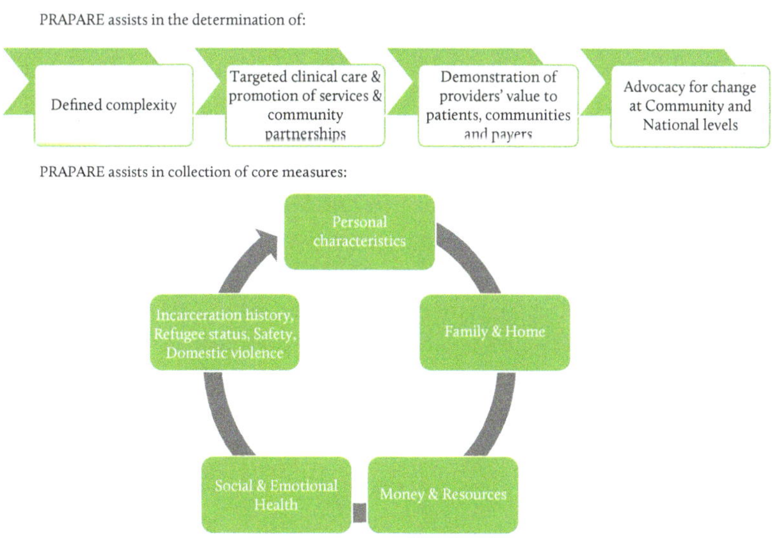

FIGURE 4.5 Prapare.

noncondescending, nonpaternalistic, or nonjudgmental approach is taken, the individual is more willing to be honest and share their concerns. This guide provides resources for assessing social determinants of health. "PRAPARE" is one example; please see Appendix 1.

One of the most well-known examples of restricted access to care was the 2014 wait time crisis that occurred in the Phoenix Veterans Administration (VA). While the Office of the Inspector General found no evidence of intentional delays in giving veterans access to care, poor management practices were uncovered (Kaboli et al., 2019). The VA conducted a 3-year study to examine the detriments of access, the impact of access on utilization, quality, and outcomes (Kaboli et al., 2019). As a result, the VA adopted a vision to address these complex and persistent issues using science, incentives, informatics, and culture to continuously improve (Kaboli et al., 2019). The VA partnered its own thought leaders with non-VA thought leaders to evaluate the results of the study, knowing that recommendations for implementation across a health system as large and as complex as the VA would be challenging. The recommendations included a combination of fee-for-service models, virtual care modalities, and face-to-face interventions as part of the VA Center for Innovations for Care and Payment. Wait times are now comparable to the private sector, but with the implementation of the Mission Act passed in 2018, priorities continue to evolve, with increased pressure to improve access within the VA (Kaboli et al., 2019).

The Health Resources and Services Administration (HRSA) within the U.S. Department of Health and Human Services is the primary agency responsible for improving access to care and systems of care for the millions of Americans geographically isolated or economically vulnerable. HRSA supports the training of health professionals and the distribution of providers where they are needed most (HRSA, 2019). HRSA developed a strategic plan for FY 2019–2022 to improve access to quality health services, develop a workforce that can meet current and future needs, and improve health equity and population health (HRSA, 2019).

The plan will operationalize and allocate resources over the 4-year period to directly support these objectives and those mandated by law. Improving access will encompass bringing quality services to underserved areas, and professionals will practice at the top of their licensure (HRSA, 2019). Innovative solutions such as telehealth will be used, and evidence-based primary care practices will be the model of care (HRSA, 2019). Access to preventative and home and

HRSA: Improving care for geographically isolated Americans and health professional training with distribution of providers in needed areas

community-based services, social supports, and care management will be implemented to connect populations to primary care and prevention (HRSA, 2019). The competencies of health care professionals will be expanded and improved to better meet the needs of populations with inadequate access (HRSA, 2019). Efforts to address professional shortages and better distribute resources will improve professional diversity (HRSA, 2019).

The Agency for Health Care Research and Quality (AHRQ) published its *National Health Care Quality Disparities Report* and identified three aims that provide guidance for improving care (AHRQ, 2018):

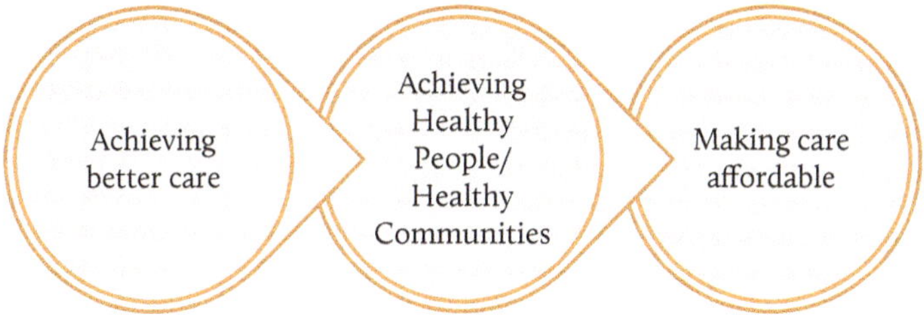
Achieving better care
Achieving Healthy People/ Healthy Communities
Making care affordable

FIGURE 4.6 Three Aims.

Better care is achieved when facilities and providers work together to expand access, enhance quality, and reduce disparities. Healthy people and communities can be achieved by addressing the leading causes of mortality and morbidity. Variations were noted by AHRQ in quality and care delivery across communities with differing race, ethnicity, and socioeconomic status (AHRQ, 2018). Making care affordable requires that health care dollars be used more wisely. Having multiple sources of reimbursement makes controlling costs more challenging (AHRQ, 2018). But delivery systems like the Patient-Centered Medical Home (PCMH) ensures health care resources are used more efficiently through improved care coordination.

"Mental illness and disorders are a major contributor to disability."

Accessing behavioral health (BH) services has been a challenge for decades. The need does not match the availability of services. The 1963 Community Mental Health Act and the good intentions to deinstitutionalize individuals with mental health disorders increased the need for services in the community (Friedman, 2017). Unfortunately, communities were not prepared and have been running to catch up ever since. One of the biggest obstacles to accessing BH services is an insufficient number of licensed BH professionals, especially in rural areas. Effective BH treatment requires a significant investment of time and effort for both the client/patient and the provider. Proven methods such as cognitive behavioral therapy (CBT) require the client/patient and provider to interact several times per month, and often, the client/patient has "homework" that needs to be reviewed by the provider (Mapanga et al., 2019). In addition, many psychotropic medications require close monitoring for side effects and improvement in symptoms, especially at treatment initiation (Mapanga et al., 2019). Transportation can be a barrier, especially if the client/patient is required to travel frequently to see a provider. Making physical office visits can be problematic for individuals who suffer from severe anxiety or paranoia or those with severe depression whose symptoms may be debilitating (Mapanga et al., 2019). And unfortunately, there still exists stigma about mental illness and treatment, even though some progress has been made in recent years.

Mental illness and disorders are a major contributor to disability (Mapanga et al., 2019). The World Health Organization notes five mental illnesses are counted in the top 20 conditions that contribute to global disease burden: anxiety disorders, major depression, schizophrenia, bipolar disorder, and dysthymia (Mapanga et al., 2019). Mental illness lacks the prioritization of medical illness; thus, inadequate resources, spending, and policies are also lacking (Mapanga et al., 2019). Low spending has contributed to a lack of neuropsychiatric facilities and even fewer resources allocated to community-based services, even though evidence demonstrates this is the most effective treatment (Mapanga et al., 2019). Community-based services ideally include a primary care provider and mental health services located in the same office. This model has been shown to be most efficient in addressing mental health and providing mental health care (Mapanga et al., 2019). The following strategies are recommended for community-based mental health care and adherence improvement (Mapanga et al., 2019):

TABLE 4.1

Cognitive Behavioral Services	Management of mental illness through links between primary care and specialty care (i.e, psychiatry, psychology)
Integrated Care	Intensified collaborative structures among an interdisciplinary team working collectively to manage all health conditions, with mental illness managed like any other chronic condition

(Continued)

TABLE 4.1 (Continued)

Task Shifting	Redistribution of nonclinical tasks to nonprofessional/ licensed staff to complete tasks that historically professionals may have performed
e-Health/ Telehealth	Use of the Internet to deliver health services and information or use of telehealth for monitoring and support
Group Therapy vs. Individual Therapy	One professional can work with several clients/patients vs. individually, reducing human resource needs
Empower Families, Caregivers, and Clients/Patients	Include family and caregivers in the treatment process, providing self-help interventions, counseling for caregiver burden, education on healthy lifestyle
Psychotherapy/ Psychosocial Interventions With or Without Medication	Treatment with psychotherapy and medication is more expensive and uses more human resources; using a multidisciplinary approach leads to better use of resources
Early Detection/ Screening	Can be conducted by the primary care practice to assess mental health issues early and implement intervention before a crisis
Systems Strategies	Adherence to clinical guidelines, continuous professional development, continuing education related to mental health

Telehealth and virtual appointments using Skype, FaceTime, Zoom, or other platforms and apps are showing promise for improving access to BH professionals and are being implemented in many areas of the United States (Mapanga et al., 2019).

Shared Decision-Making

Shared decision-making (SDM) is a process for clients/patients, medical providers, and other stakeholders to participate in medical decisions and are thought to improve client/patient and health system outcomes (Groot, Waldron, Carr, McMullen, & Bandura, 2017). This model or process focuses on the relationship between a client/patient and provider to make mutually agreeable treatment decisions. SDM supports the ethical principle of autonomy by encouraging an interactive provider–patient relationship, discussion of client/patient preferences, and arrival at mutual consensus (Groot, Waldron, Carr, McMullen, & Bandura, 2017).

SDM has demonstrated evidence that it improves the quality of care and client/patient knowledge and participation, especially for those who are socioeconomically disadvantaged and those with complex chronic illnesses (Groot, Waldron, Carr, McMullen, & Bandura, 2017). Participation and shared decisions in care result in improved adherence.

A well-cited SDM model, the Interpersonal Shared Decision-Making Model (IP-SDM), is directed to all individuals involved in a client's/patient's care outside the physician relationship (Garvelink et al., 2018). The IP-SDM addresses the individual, the health care team, and the policy/context (Garvelink et al., 2018). The model was validated in 2011 and has been adopted in multiple care settings (Garvelink et al., 2018). Other SDM models include the OPTION model, the Three-Talk Model, and the Ecological Model, but there is little evidence to support their efficacy in the literature. Groot et al. recently published their intent to produce a framework using the IP-SDM to even more clearly define the implementation of SDM and to test, confirm, and refine the framework to improve quality of care and increase efficiencies in health care systems. Even though there are no well-studied frameworks or clear direction for SDM, familiarity with the IP-SDM can assist in helping clients/patients to participate in their care.

The IP-SDM framework guides the process for sharing decisions (Groot, Waldron, Carr, McMullen, & Bandura, 2017):

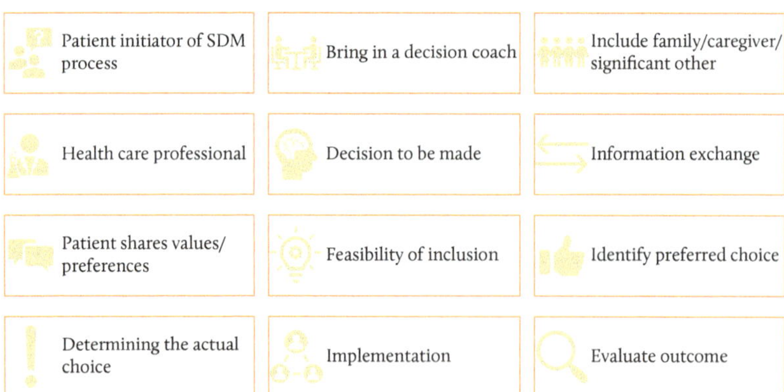
Patient initiator of SDM process
Bring in a decision coach
Include family/caregiver/ significant other
Health care professional
Decision to be made
Information exchange
Patient shares values/ preferences
Feasibility of inclusion
Identify preferred choice
Determining the actual choice
Implementation
Evaluate outcome

FIGURE 4.7 Process for Sharing Decisions.

A method for evaluating client engagement and ability to participate in shared decision-making is to use the Patient Activation Measure (PAM). The PAM measures the level to which an individual is engaged in their care. Researchers Justin Hibbard, Jean Stockard, Eldon Mahoney, and Martin Tusler created this tool that defines patient activation and characteristics (Heath, 2017):

Patient Activation Measure	
Definition and characteristics	1. The ability to self-manage illness and other problems 2. The ability to engage in activities that reduce worsening health and activities that maintain health 3. The ability to be involved in treatment and diagnostic choices 4. The ability to collaborate with providers 5. The ability to select providers and provider organizations based on quality and performance 6. The ability to navigate the health system and act
Four levels of activation	1. A belief that a patient's active role in health is important 2. Having the confidence and knowledge to make decisions 3. Taking proactive action to improve and maintain health 4. Staying motivated and active even when under stress

The PAM has 22 items that align these four levels of activation. It has been shown to be highly reliable for measuring activation and for the design of individual care plans (Heath, 2017). It can also be used for large-scale programs to determine the effectiveness of efforts to improve patient participation by administering it before and after any interventions. Hibbard et al. also created a shorter version of the PAM using 13 items instead of 22. The shorter version is meant to reduce the time needed to conduct the measure, especially in the clinical setting, but it yields the same results (Heath, 2017). The 13-item survey still covers the four levels of activation, and the accuracy rate is 92% (Heath, 2017). The PAM is licensed by Insignia Health and therefore requires the purchase of the rights to use it in practice. The American Medical Group Association recommends conducting the PAM with all new patients, whether that means using a paper survey or integrating the survey into an EHR (Heath, 2017).

We know health care is not "one size fits all," and using a tool like the PAM can help support the goal of patient-centered care by improving patient participation. Having knowledge of an individual's understanding, skills, beliefs, and motivations will support appropriate and comprehensive care coordination (Heath, 2017). Appendix 4 provides an example of a scored PAM with information on licensure.

- Level 1: Disengaged and overwhelmed
- Level 2: Becoming aware but still struggling
- Level 3: Taking action
- Level 4: Maintaining behaviors and pushing further

FIGURE 4.8 The Patient Activation Measure (PAM).

The Impact of Time on Shared Decision-Making (SDM)

Time is the greatest barrier to SDM. Time is a necessary resource for clients/patients and providers to collaborate, and when it is constrained, SDM is nearly impossible. During a scheduled client/patient encounter, planning for what will be discussed is essential for success. For bedside encounters and unplanned office encounters, there is a need to improvise so the needed time for discussion is included.

SDM is sometimes viewed as a "nice thing to do" rather than something required for client/patient–provider encounters. To make SDM routinely part of health encounters, clinicians need to learn and appreciate what is concerning the client/patient and what is important to them. By the same token, clients/patients cannot assume clinicians understand their situations without having conversations. Clinicians need to learn and appreciate their clients'/patients' priorities and then negotiate through them to achieve high-quality care (Pieterse, 2019). Clinicians need to be as comfortable asking questions as they are at providing answers. Clients/patients should take time to reflect on what clinicians share. Clinicians need to make more time to sit down, make eye contact, and give patients their undivided attention, demonstrating to the clients/patients that "this is your time."

These are attitudes and practices not currently consistent in health care culture (Pieterse, 2019). Changing these attitudes and practices will go a long way to successful SDM, but time remains the barrier. Science needs to be applied to develop scheduling algorithms that can accommodate these types of encounters (Pieterse, 2019). It is not necessary to conduct such encounters face to face: other methods such as virtual encounters can be just as effective (Pieterse, 2019). Even if we see practices evolve to support improving encounters, policymakers must play a role by understanding the value of optimizing time and access to providers through development of policy and reimbursement structures that support meaningful time in care delivery (Pieterse, 2019).

Adherence Incentives

Peer participation and support are the most effective means of sustaining better health outcomes from wellness activities (Volpp, 2018). According to Volpp and Mohota in their *NEJM Catalyst* report, "What Creates Behavior Change May Not Sustain It," peer support used in addition to financial gains seem to be the most successful of incentives (Volpp, 2018). But Volpp and Mohota also report that wellness programs are "worthless" unless followed with properly funded medical care from a provider (Volpp, 2018). Employers and insurers have been using financial rewards and penalties for some time, with mixed results (Wong, 2019). To improve on this, a combination of financial and social approaches is needed (Wong, 2019).

"... family and friend support are the most important."

A survey conducted in January 2019 revealed that individuals see family and friend support as the most important in realizing patient goals, with education, clinician support, and financial rewards following nearly equally in importance (Wong, 2019).

Dr. Charlene Wong, an adolescent medical pediatrician, expresses concerns about financial incentives when using these as extrinsic factors because they interfere with intrinsic motivation, which is more sustainable for behavior change (Wong, 2019). Studies have shown that individuals change behaviors as long as the

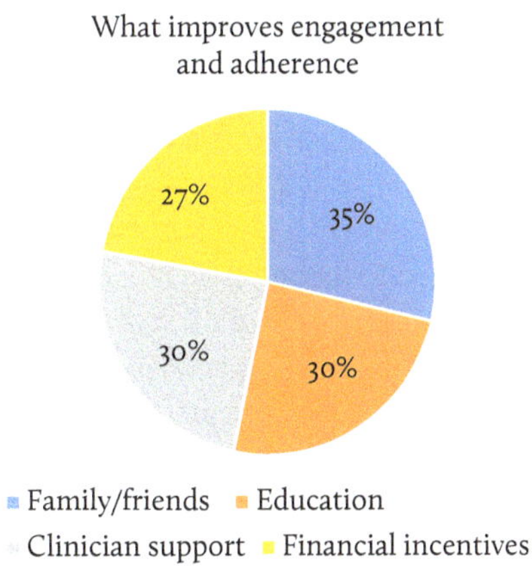

FIGURE 4.9 What Improves Engagement and Adherence.

financial incentive is available, but once removed, the effect diminishes rather quickly (Wong, 2019). Approaches rooted in social support have a more long-lasting impact because, in theory, family and friends are seen as a permanent presence in an individual's life (Wong, 2019).

Financial penalties for lack of behavior change are concerning, says Dr. Namita Mohota, an internal medicine physician (Wong, 2019). She asserts that penalties are especially harmful to vulnerable populations, further marginalizing and exacerbating health inequities (Wong, 2019). Financial incentives appear to be the most effective for patient engagement and risk reduction for things like smoking cessation, completing preventative screenings, healthy eating, and fitness (Wong, 2019). Dr. Wong believes improved and sustained adherence can be achieved when social supports are combined with financial incentives (Wong, 2019).

Conclusion

The reasons an individual adheres to prescribed medication or treatment can vary but are not typical because the individual is just "difficult." As case managers, we need to make every effort to learn and understand the challenges our clients/patients face. We need to "listen to their voice," truly hear them, and, once we have learned what is important, negotiate how health improvements might occur. Lack of adherence is costly, so the time and effort expended to improve adherence will result in a positive return on investment.

A significant contributor to poor adherence is a lack of or poor access to quality care and services. Even though more individuals are reported to have health coverage, the number engaged with primary care providers (PCP) has not kept pace. Case managers should help facilitate the connection with a PCP but also support the development of a trusted relationship for better engagement. Improving access to care also involves addressing determinants to access with tools and suggestions provided in this chapter. Of special interest is access to behavioral health services with some resources on how to improve access in an era when resources can be scarce.

For clients/patients to be engaged in their health, they must also be included in decisions related to diagnostics and treatment. We have examined SDM, a framework for participation, and other tools that help evaluate how engagement or the potential for engagement can be determined. We also know and understand the most desired resource is time, but time has yet to be elevated to a must-have for improved engagement. We also examined the benefits and detriments of incentives and disincentives to improve adherence, learning that social support far outweighs financial penalties when trying to motivate individuals to change behaviors.

In the next chapter, we will examine the role of care coordination and transitions of care in improving adherence.

Putting It Into Practice

Ask yourself these questions and reflect to target interventions for improving adherence:

- Do you understand what impacts engagement? Do you observe the presence of these in your patient's environment? The following list provides examples of and interventions to improve engagement:
  - An individual's engagement capacity influences their behaviors
  - If care is patient-centered, engagement improves
  - Patient engagement leads to patient satisfaction
  - Measure patient satisfaction as an outcome
  - Patients are consumers of health care and expect similar experiences to other businesses
  - Examine what is preventing satisfactory care: access, cost, geography, delays, or disparities due to race, gender, age, ethnicity, or socioeconomic status
  - Use tools to assess and address SDOH
  - Establish resources in your community to address SDOH
  - Facilitate out-of-the-box mental health treatment: telehealth, virtual visits, and community-based services, and encourage early screening
  - Support SDM: assess a patient's ability to participate and then provide interventions to assist
  - Explore the potential use of incentives for adherence, but avoid use of penalties

References

Agency for Health Care Research and Quality. (2018). *Overview of quality and access in the U.S. health care system.* Rockville, MD: Agency for Health Care Research and Quality. https://www.ahrq.gov/research/findings/nhqrdr/nhqdr16/overview.html

Angove, R., & Boselovic, J. A. (2018). Complementary approaches to patient engagement in patient-centered outcomes research. *NEJM Catalyst,* 1–6.

Das, L. T., Abramson, E., & Kaushal, R. (2019). High-need, high-cost patients offer solutions for improving their care and reducing costs. *NEJM Catalyst.* https://catalyst.nejm.org/high-need-high-cost-patients-solutions/?utm_campaign=Connect%20Weekly&utm_source=hs_email&utm_medium=email&utm_content=79017922&_hsenc=p2ANqtz-9OuT92ibupyJ_c6XT-bUI2zrBCbyWLu_IUTbUGDt8fHkWKK1Yho9yKhonaxDpo8q6atBAu1Jh-FWak1wGHzd919D

Friedman, J. (2017, July 1). Improving access to care via telebehavioral health. *Health Management Technology-Digital.*

Garvelink, M. M., Groen-van de Ven, L., Smits, C., Franken, R., Dassen-Vernooij, M., & Légaré, F. (2018). Shared decision making about housing transitions for persons with dementia: A four-case care network perspective. *The Gerontologist.* doi:https://doi.org/10.1093%2Fgeront%2Fgny073

Groot, G., Waldron, T., Carr, T., McMullen, L., & Bandura, L. A. (2017). Development of a program theory for shared decision-making: A realist review protocol. *Systematic Reviews, 6*(114), 1–9. doi:10.1186/s13643-017-0508-5

Heath, S. (2017, September 12). *What is the patient activation measure in patient-centered care?* PatientEngagementHIT. https://patientengagementhit.com/news/what-is-the-patient-activation-measure-in-patient-centered-care

Health Resources and Services Administration. (2019). *Healthy communities, healthy people: Strategic plan 2019–2022.* Washington, DC: Health Resources and Services Administration.

Hsiang, W., Lukasiewicz, A., Gentry, M., Kim, C., Leslie, M., Pelker, R., … & Wiznia, D. (2019). Medicaid patients have greater difficulty scheduling health care appointments compared with private insurance patients: A meta-analysis. *The Journal of Health Care Organization, Provision, and Financing, 56,* 1–9. doi:10.1177/0046958019838118

Kaboli, P., Miake-Lye, I., Ruser, C., Yano, E., Orshansky, G., Rubenstein, L., … & Hempel, S. (2019). Sequelae of an evidence-based approach to management for access to care in the Veterans Health Administration. *Medical Care, 57*(10), S213–S220.

Mapanga, W., Casteleijn, D., Ramiah, C., Odendaa, W., Metu, Z., Robertson, D., & Goudge, J. (2019). Strategies to strengthen the provision of mental health care at the primary care setting: An evidence map. *PLOS ONE, 14*(9), 1–15. doi:https://doi.org/10.1371/journal.pone.0222162

Office of Disease Prevention and Health Promotion. (2019, November). *Access to health services.* Healthy People 2020. https://www.healthypeople.gov/2020/topics-objectives/topic/Access-to-Health-Services

Pieterse, A. S. (2019). Shared decision-making and the importance of time. *Journal of the American Medical Association, 322*(1), 25–26.

Ransco, M. (2019). Patient experience. *NEJM Catalyst Innovations in Care Delivery.*

Sieck, C., Walker, D., & Retchin, S. (2019). The patient engagement capacity model: What factors determine a patient's ability to engage? *NEJM Catalyst,* 1–7.

Spruce, L. (2019). Back to basics: Social determinants of health. *AORN.* doi:http://doi.org/10.1002/aorn.12722

Volpp, K. G. (2018). *Patient engagement survey: What creates behavior change may not sustain it.* Waltham, MA: *NEJM Catalyst Innovations in Care Delivery.*

Wagle, N. (2019). Taxonomy of the patient voice. *NEJM Catalyst Innovations in Care Delivery,* 1–4.

Wong, C. (2019). Why no single health incentive works. *NEJM Catalyst Innovations in Care Delivery.*

Figure Credits

Fig. 4.1: Source: https://catalyst.nejm.org/doi/full/10.1056/CAT.19.0001.

Fig 4.3: Lala Tanmoy Das, Erika L. Abramson, and Rainu Kaushal, "What High-Need High-Cost Patients Say About How to Reduce High Utilization of ED and Inpatient Services, from 'High-Need, High-Cost Patients Offer Solutions for Improving Their Care and Reducing Costs,'" NEJM Catalyst. Copyright © 2019 by Massachusetts Medical Society.

Fig. 4.3a: Copyright © 2015 Depositphotos/kaer_dstock.

Fig. 4.3b: Copyright © 2015 Depositphotos/VisualGeneration.

Fig. 4.9: Source: https://catalyst.nejm.org/doi/full/10.1056/CAT.19.0667.

5

Care Coordination and Care Transitions to Support Adherence

The Vital Role of Outpatient Care

Most health care costs lie with a small percentage of the population, and a reasonable strategy to address these costs is to target efforts on this sector. High utilizers are typically older, have multiple chronic conditions, and are admitted more frequently (Lee, Whitman, Vakharia, & Taksler, 2016). To reduce utilization, improvements are needed in care coordination, adherence to medication, self-management, patient–physician communication, and meeting social needs. A percentage of high utilizers may have efficient care coordination, but they are challenged with conditions that are expensive to treat—for example, cancer. Others who may benefit from more aggressive care coordination efforts are those with social and behavioral challenges (Lee, Whitman, Vakharia, & Taksler, 2016). For individuals who have had episodes of critical illness, coordination of intensive services and transition management are required to prevent delays in transitions from the ICU to the medical floor and, ultimately, discharge to outpatient care (Lee, Whitman, Vakharia, & Taksler, 2016).

When working with clients/patients frequently admitted to the hospital or emergency department, outpatient management must first focus on establishing a trusted relationship to engage the client/patient better, target disease control, evaluate for psychiatric/behavioral interventions, and provide social supports. If the client/patient does not have a relationship with a primary care provider (PCP), this would be the priority.

Clients/patients with complexity often do well in medical home environments or integrated primary care practices.

"Siloed care results in missed opportunities, gaps in care, and errors that create risk for readmission."

Many facets of our health care system continue to operate in silos, or without interdisciplinary collaboration, focusing primarily on specific diseases or conditions (Swan, 2019). Individuals with multiple chronic conditions have unique needs and transition often between settings and providers. Siloed care results in missed opportunities, gaps in care, and errors that create risk for adverse events. Poor communication and care coordination during transitions perpetuate risk. Add to that a lack of shared information with the client/patient for risk of adverse events, poor care quality, admissions, and readmissions (Swan et al., 2019). Nearly 50% of clients/patients experience at least one medical error post-discharge, and one in five clients/patients experience an adverse event post-discharge (Swan et al., 2019). Improving communication among and between providers could prevent one-half of these events (Swan et al., 2019). One in five Medicare beneficiaries discharged from the hospital is readmitted within 30 days, and 34% are readmitted within 90 days (Swan, Haas, & Conway-Phillips, 2019).

Haas et al. developed a care model with registered nurses in 2013 that enhances quality and cost-effectiveness through care coordination (Hass et al., 2019). The Care Coordination and Transition Management model (CCTM) is a framework that includes these nine dimensions (Haas et al., 2019):

1. Support for self-management
2. Education and engagement with individuals and families
3. Coaching and counseling of individuals and families
4. Advocacy
5. Population health management
6. Teamwork and collaboration
7. Cross-setting communication and transition
8. Person-centered care planning
9. Nursing process

The CCTM model has the potential to guide acute care practice and discharge teaching and planning, facilitate care transitions between providers and settings, and provide support so individuals with multiple chronic conditions can stay in their homes, reside in assisted living settings, or receive care in the home from community resources to self-manage their health (Haas et al., 2019).

In 2013, the Centers for Medicare and Medicaid (CMS) urged states to implement care coordination programs to improve access to primary care (Capp et al., 2017). Many programs were developed by hospitals and focused on emergency department (ED) care coordination whereby appointments were facilitated, referrals to address social determinants of health were made, and care plans were developed, but there was little to no community involvement (Capp et al., 2017). The results of these programs have been mixed, with a lack of primary care engagement and no involvement of behavioral health or health coaching (Capp et al., 2017).

"More than one-half of all hospital admissions originate with a visit to the ED."

Community-based primary care that includes care coordination and multidisciplinary community-based programs have been shown to reduce ED use and hospital admissions and increase primary care visits (Capp et al., 2017). More than one-half of all hospital admissions originate with a visit to the ED, and one in five previously hospitalized patients return to the ED within 30 days, with one-half of those being readmitted (Capp et al., 2017). Typically, ED care does not include any form of prevention or disease management, but an ED program that includes follow-up after the ED with facilitation of a PCP appointment and follow-up for 180 days supports the reduction of ED use and hospitalization (Capp et al., 2017). Multidisciplinary primary care coordination utilizing community resources also prevents this utilization by populations with multiple chronic conditions (Capp et al., 2017). Research related to these programs reinforces follow-up as essential to comprehensive care and sustained reduction in ED use and admissions (Capp et al., 2017).

Clients/patients receiving care in multiple settings are often the victims of poor communication because of existing fragmentation. Improving care coordination and transition management throughout the continuum of care is the answer (Roach, 2019). Establishing methods and processes to communicate effectively across and between settings and providers should be standardized (Roach, 2019). Much work is still required to create and implement such processes. Case managers are well positioned to coordinate care and manage transitions across the continuum, especially for those with complex care needs. Individuals over the age of 65 or younger people with complex health conditions are more likely to be transferred between facilities and to receive care from multiple providers. Integral to success is the leadership role of the case manager working with an interdisciplinary team. The case manager leading a care transition enhances continuity by communicating with all stakeholders (client/patient/family, receiving provider, and PCP), educating and coaching the client/patient/family about the transition plan and how best to self-manage during the various transition points, and assisting the client/patient/family with navigating the health care system (i.e., making and keeping appointments; Jeffs et al., 2018). The care coordination process is more effectively managed when a single point of contact collaborates with other health care professionals to prepare the client/patient/family for transitions and coordination of needs. Interdisciplinary collaboration ensures seamless transitions, especially for older, more complex clients/patients.

Supporting Outpatient Care

Well-coordinated outpatient care has been shown to result in a 15–50% reduction in health care costs (Zulman, 2019). These results occur when clients/patients are engaged with primary care providers. As discussed earlier in this guide, the most common barriers to client/patient engagement include chronic conditions with debilitating symptoms, mental illness, fragmented care across providers and systems, isolation and lack of social support, financial insecurity, and unsafe environments. When these social determinants are addressed with communication, referrals to services, and activities that foster trust, client/patient engagement improves. Whether these barriers are addressed as part of comprehensive primary care or a multidisciplinary approach, patient-centered care is achieved.

Many health conditions can be managed well in the outpatient setting, primarily if outpatient care is supported with comprehensive care coordination activities, such as greater availability of extended appointment times, coaching for chronic condition management, home health, telehealth, transportation to medical appointments, housing, and employment resources. If a primary care practice does not offer comprehensive care coordination services, an interdisciplinary collaboration can be established with a case manager to coordinate care with community resources and outside providers. The following are examples of specific strategies case managers can implement to facilitate better outpatient engagement (Zulman, 2019).

TABLE 5.1

Assist the client/patient in scheduling multiple appointments in one day to minimize risk of missing an appointment
Reduce care fragmentation by accessing medical records, facilitating interdisciplinary meetings to discuss the needs of complex clients/patients, and communicating with specialists on behalf of the client/patient
Assist with finding transportation resources, such as bus passes, taxi vouchers, and non-emergent medical transportation
Offer video/telephone appointments for follow-up
Offer home visits for follow-up
Address health literacy by graphically labeling medications and coaching on appropriate use
Review metric readings with the client/patient (e.g., blood pressure, blood sugar)
Connect clients/patients to financial resources, such as affordable housing, food banks/food stamps, utility assistance, pharmacy scholarships, and discount programs; work with pharmacists for generic formulations or simplification to reduce out-of-pocket expenses
Temporarily take over some of the coordination activities performed by the caregiver to reduce caregiver burden
Provide phone numbers for quicker access to providers, not a central operator
Integrate behavioral health care into the medical care plan
Help clients/patients prioritize social demands and provide resources to reduce risk as a result of poor social support
Begin to build trust by meeting the client/patient where they live, during an outpatient appointment, or while confined in the hospital
Accept that substance use may be a constant challenge
Assist the client/patient with finding a mental health provider
Determine what is essential to the client/patient and validate it as a priority
Be present during encounters to assist with understanding or helping the client/patient prepare for appointments with questions to ask
For clients/patients with low health literacy levels, make self-management classes available or refer to a nutritionist or other appropriate ancillary support
Help clients/patients identify their strengths and the challenges that impact their ability to self-manage. Coach them in targeted solutions and facilitate mental health counseling to build insight if warranted
Determine what motivates the client/patient and what their goals are so engagement can be maintained

Supporting Outpatient Care with Telehealth

The recent COVID-19 pandemic and associated shelter-in-place mandates resulted in a decrease in engagement with routine medical care. For individuals with chronic conditions, a loss of connection with providers can mean the difference between condition control and an increase in symptoms, poor condition control, and hospitalization.

While not widely adopted until recently, telehealth became a viable option for individuals to stay connected with their providers and for support and monitoring of their conditions. With rapid adoption and deployment of telehealth due to the COVID-19 pandemic, another concern came to light, and that was reimbursement. One of the reasons telehealth had been slow to implement was reimbursement and payment structures. The pandemic and the need to ensure continuity of care for outpatient management of health resulted in the Centers for Medicare and Medicaid and other payers to quickly adopt and implement payment structures.

Telehealth had originally been developed to bridge geographic disparities and to supplement mental health services due to provider shortages and limitations. The need for clients/patients to receive care without exposing them to a dangerous virus has catapulted this technology and care delivery model as a new standard.

For some clients/patients, telehealth may become a preference; for others, it may not seem to provide the level of comfort and satisfaction typically experienced with in-person visits with their clinicians. A shift in communication strategies may be required for providers to engage clients/patients and to ensure that they feel heard and understood.

According to a telehealth blog published by the University of Arizona, providers need to develop "screenside manners," which are akin to bedside manners (Heath, 2020). As with in-person encounters, the provider or clinician should follow these guidelines for telehealth visits (Heath, 2017):

1. Look the part
    a. Present yourself in a professional manner
    b. "Wear the white coat"
2. Use body language and physical cues
    a. Mirror body language and physical reactions to those of in-person interactions

   b. Look at the computer camera, not the screen
   c. Make sure there are no distractions in your space
   d. Do not spend the entire encounter taking notes
3. Be prepared
   a. Review the client's/patient's history, chart, file
   b. Be prepared for any technical glitches; know who to call for assistance; know how to assist the client/patient with troubleshooting
4. Establish rapport
   a. While challenging, do your best to convey warmth and empathy
   b. By looking into the camera and not at the screen, it appears to the person on the receiving end that you are looking at them. If you look at the screen, it appears you are looking down.
   c. What and how the clinician communicates is of the highest importance. This is the way to ensure the client/patient experiences empathy and feels like they are the focus; this will foster a positive encounter.
   d. Ask questions at appropriate intervals and explain if you need to take notes

Implementing these practices will ensure that telehealth encounters are successful and patient satisfaction is maintained. Please see Appendix 17 for telehealth resources.

Elements That Support Engagement Using Interdisciplinary Teams

Client/patient engagement is further supported by the interdisciplinary team members who may be involved in their care. The varying disciplines help each other see the client/patient through a different lens and from a less familiar perspective. Members of the team need not all be professional; based on the population served, the team may be well served by including non-clinical staff who have experienced challenges similar to the population: for example, substance use, homelessness, or needing a native speaker for an ethnic group included in the population. The following are elements that support engagement using interdisciplinary teams (Zulman, 2019):

1. Develop teams with diverse professional backgrounds that match client/patient needs: mental health, cardiology, endocrinology, pharmacy, etc.
2. Hire staff who speak languages other than English to facilitate communication with non-English-speaking clients/patients
3. Hold regular interprofessional/interdisciplinary meetings to assess client/patient progress and to address the challenges of team members to prevent burnout

Skill Sets for Interdisciplinary Teams

Necessary skill sets or training to impart to members of an interdisciplinary team are emotional intelligence and motivational interviewing. These skill sets improve the ability to recognize in any individual what is essential or preferred, their strengths, and challenges for self-management, and provide coaching for problem-solving strategies. Resources for expanding the case manager's emotional intelligence and motivational interviewing skills can be found in the appendices of this guide. See Appendix 6 and Appendix 7.

These and other strategies recommended for client/patient engagement are not without challenges. How do the case manager and interdisciplinary team members handle dysfunctional engagement behaviors? Sometimes clients/patients engage with one discipline but not with others: for example, an individual who only engages with social services but not the case manager to learn how to better self-manage diabetes. A patient-centered approach is not forfeited when these behaviors are addressed, if done correctly. The case manager can coach and provide information to the social worker to help the client/patient better manage diabetes but should also make sure they understand where the information is originating. To expand on this example, an individual may demand an unsustainable level of resources. In such a case, all team members must be clear and united in their approach: "We will teach *you* how to problem-solve and give *you* support, but we will not do everything for you." Another example is the individual who engages with multiple community resources: the result is the agencies begin tripping over one another, services may be duplicated, and the client/patient is overutilizing resources without changing behaviors. In such a case, steps must be taken to bring representatives from all the agencies together to collaborate on what each can bring to the patient to prevent duplication or overburdening any one agency.

Preventing Admissions and Readmissions

Clients/patients engaged in outpatient care who follow treatment recommendations, keep appointments, and take medications as prescribed are less likely to be admitted to the hospital with symptom exacerbations and complications. For those with complex or multiple chronic conditions, the risk of admission is higher even if they are engaged in outpatient care. However, the number of admissions, readmissions, and ED visits can be reduced with effective care coordination and transition management. To prevent admissions, we must shift the focus from the acute care episode to the continuum of care.

Before a client/patient is discharged, the level of risk for readmission should be assessed. A tool available in the public domain that is a quick and easy determinant of readmission is the LACE tool. The LACE tool, or index, as it is sometimes known, assesses length of stay, acuity of admission, presence of comorbidities, and history of ED visits. Each element is scored, and the higher the score, the greater the risk of readmission, especially within 30 days. The length-of-stay score is applied based on days confined: for 1 to 3 days, a score of 1 to 3 is applied; for 4 to 6 days, a score of 4 is applied; 7 to 13 days receive a 5, and 14 or more days is a 7. The acuity score is based on whether the admission originated in the ED; if so, a score of 3 is applied. For comorbidities, cardiovascular disease, a history of MI, peripheral vascular disease, or diabetes without complications receives a score of 1 for each that is present; a score of 2 is applied for COPD, liver or renal disease, or any tumor, leukemia, or lymphoma; 3 points are given for dementia or connective tissue disease; 4 points are given for AIDS or moderate to severe renal or liver disease; and 6 points are given for any metastatic disease. The final element scored addresses the number of ED visits in the previous 6 months, and if any ED visits have occurred, a score of 4 is applied. If the total number of points is greater than or equal to 10, the patient/client is at high risk for readmission. A copy of the LACE tool can be found in the appendices of this guide as Appendix 8.

Clients/patients at high risk for readmission require additional assessment to determine what or where vulnerabilities exist. Assess the presence of social determinants, such as the inability to attend appointments, the presence of social support, financial challenges, low health literacy, or behavioral conditions. The presence of these or other barriers increases risk for admission and worsening health, and strategies to reduce risk need to be developed as part of transition management and care coordination. Key to the success of any transition plan is to include the client/patient and their support system, provide coaching in self-management, ensure a post-discharge appointment has been scheduled and the client/patient has the means to keep the appointment, communicate the plan to all clinicians involved in the client/patient's care, and verify that any community resources are in place.

Follow-up post-discharge should occur in 48 hours to verify that the client/patient has their needs met: medications, services, social supports, confirmation of a follow-up visit, and a means to keep the appointment. For those at high risk of readmission, the case manager should follow up with the client/patient after the visit for any changes in medication or treatment and then set a schedule for regular contact so any changes in condition can be addressed expeditiously.

Clients/patients engaged in outpatient care who follow treatment recommendations, keep appointments, and take medications as prescribed are less likely to be admitted to the hospital.

The term "care transition" is used synonymously with discharge, but in actuality, care transitions are an ongoing process, not just the act of moving a client/patient from one setting to another. Providing a client/patient, especially one challenged with complex health conditions, with written instructions, prescriptions to fill, and a phone number to call for an appointment is not a care transition. There are transition models that include 30- to 90-day follow-up; some include interdisciplinary teams with patient/client access to health coaches, pharmacists, nurse case managers, and social workers in addition to their PCPs. Interdisciplinary team management has been shown to improve outcomes because of the diverse clinical knowledge and expertise that an interdisciplinary team offers (Schentrup, 2019).

Improving client/patient self-management is the goal of any case/care management program. The ability to discharge a patient from CM services because they can manage their condition is the most significant outcome and measure of success. One of the strategies of self-management is the ability to engage with providers, but many of our clients/patients do not know how to do this, so we must coach them. If the CM can attend appointments with them, this is an excellent way to start the process to give them support and encouragement, but not to the extent that they are enabled. You must begin to teach them what to do and what to ask at medical appointments so that they can begin to take control of their health.

"Ask Me Three" is a well-recognized tool designed by health literacy experts to help patients become more engaged with providers (IHI, 2020). The CM begins by coaching the client/patient on how to ask (IHI, 2020):

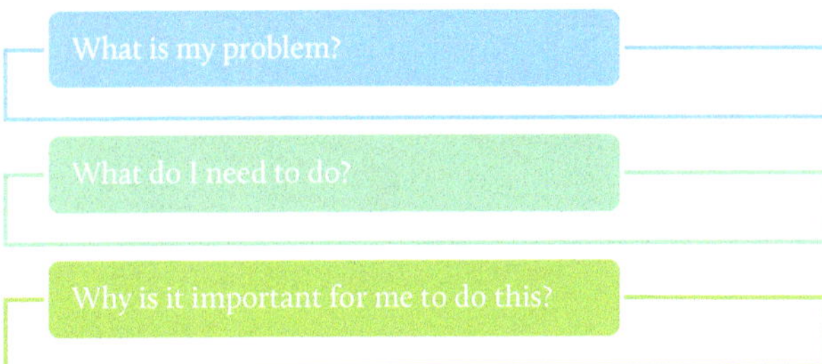

FIGURE 5.1 Ask Me Three.

The recommended coaching includes practicing with your client/patient using teach-back to prepare them for the appointment and to follow up immediately after to see how things went. More information about "Ask Me Three" can be found in Appendix 9.

The 2010 Patient Protection and Affordable Care Act, Title V, defined health literacy as "the degree to which an individual has the capacity to obtain, communicate, process, and understand basic health information and services to make appropriate health decisions" (CDC, 2019). Everyone needs information they can understand to make informed decisions, especially when it comes to health. Health literacy is vital to everyone because at some point in their life, they will need to understand and use health information. Health literacy is not just important when seeing a doctor or when in the hospital but also in everyday life to make good decisions about preventing health problems.

Even individuals who are highly educated or well-read may be uncomfortable with medical terms or unfamiliar with how the human body functions. We, as health care professionals, need to be cognizant of how we present information—we must make it easy to understand and allow the individual to feel comfortable enough to ask questions. When we share information, especially any written information, we should make it accurate, accessible, and actionable (CDC, 2019).

- Accurate
    - Does not mean "dumbing down"
    - Factual but understandable
- Accessible
    - Have the main message
    - Make available in multiple locations and formats
    - Easy to read, brief
    - Available in appropriate languages
    - Visually appealing
- Actionable
    - With the information provided, give suggestions for something that *can* be done

"Care transitions are an ongoing process, not just the act of moving a patient from one level of care to another."

Health Literacy Toolshed www.healthliteracy.bu.edu/

The REALM-SF is a very brief health literacy assessment endorsed by the Agency for Health Care Research and Quality (AHRQ), and it was revised in 2016. The assessment can be found in the appendices as Appendix 10. Additional health literacy tools that are disease-specific and in other languages can be accessed from the Health Literacy Toolshed at https://healthliteracy.bu.edu/all. Poor health literacy is a determinant that impacts all aspects of an individual's health and should be assessed early in the CM process.

Conclusion

Adherence occurs when self-management is supported. As case managers, we must support outpatient care and provide the tools necessary for self-management. In the next chapter, we will focus on medication adherence. This is where the adherence movement and CMAG started, but as you can see, medication is now just part of the adherence equation, albeit a crucial part.

Putting It Into Practice

Ask yourself these questions and reflect to target interventions for improving patient engagement in outpatient care to support adherence:

- How do case managers support patient engagement in primary care?
- How do you assist patients with multiple admissions and ED visits, establish a trusted relationship with a PCP?
- Communication with and among the patient's providers is key to well-coordinated care—Are you, the case manager, prepared to be the facilitator of this communication?
- How will you improve care coordination and care transitions to prevent admissions and readmissions, especially for vulnerable populations?
- Does your organization provide care coordination and transition programs from the ED to outpatient practices?
- Case managers leading interdisciplinary teams is a more effective process for care coordination and transitions. Do case managers lead your interdisciplinary teams?
- How will you facilitate well-coordinated outpatient care to reduce health care costs ?
- Would you consider implementing the strategies outlined by Zulman to improve engagement?
- Have you committed to familiarizing yourself with Telehealth Guidelines?
- Will you incorporate Ask Me 3 in your patient education to improve patient-provider engagement?
- Do you feel prepared to address health literacy issues with accurate, accessible, and actionable patient information?
- How can you incorporate tools and resources to assess and address levels of health literacy?

References

Agency for Health Care Research and Quality. (2016, February). *Health literacy measurement tools (revised).* Retrieved from https://www.ahrq.gov/health-literacy/quality-resources/tools/literacy/index.html

Capp, R., Misky, G., Lindrooth, R., Honigman, B., Logan, H., Hardy, R., & Nguyen, D. (2017). Coordination program reduced acute care use and increased primary care visits among frequent emergency care users. *Health Affairs, 36*(10), 1705–1711. doi:10.1377/hlthaff.2017.0612

Centers for Disease Control and Prevention. (2019, October 23). *What is health literacy?* Retrieved from www.cdc.gov/healthliteracy/learn.index.html/

Haas, S., Swan, B., Start, R., Conway-Phillips, R., & de la Pena, L. (2019). Developing a business case for the care coordination and transition management model: Need, methods, and measures. *Nursing Economics, 37*(3), 118–125.

Heath, S. (2020, April 9). *Communication tips for a good telehealth patient experience.* Retrieved from https://patientengagementhit.com

Institutes for Health Care Improvement. (2020). *Ask me 3: Good questions for your good health.* Retrieved from http://www.ihi.org/resources/Pages/Tools/Ask-Me-3-Good-Questions-for-Your-Good-Health.aspx

Jeffs, L., Saragosa, M., Law, M., Kuluski, K., Espin, S., & Parker, H. (2018). The varying roles of nurses during interfacility care transitions. *Journal of Nursing Care Quality, 33*(1), E1–E6. doi:10.1097/NCQ.0000000000000248

Lee, N., Whitman, N., Vakharia, N., & Taksler, G. (2016). High-cost patients: Hot-spotters don't explain the half of it. *Journal of General Internal Medicine, 32*(1), 28–34. doi:10.1007/s11606-016-3790-3

Naqvi, S. (2016, April 13). *Using LACE as a tool to avoid unnecessary hospital readmissions.* Retrieved from https://www.allscripts.com/2016/04/using-lace-as-a-tool-to-avoid-unnecessary-hospital-readmissions/

Roach, A. (2019). An academic-practice partnership: fostering collaboration and improving care across settings. *Nurse Educator, 44*(2), 98–101. doi:10.1097/NNE.0000000000000557

Schentrup, D. B. (2019). Interprofessional teams: Lessons learned from a nurse-led clinic. *The Journal for Nurse Practitioners, 15*, 331–335. doi:https://doi.org/10.1016/j.nurpra.2019.02.016

Swan, B. H. (2019, November/December). Care coordination: Roles of registered nurses across the care continuum. *Nursing Economics, 37*(6), 317–323.

Swan, B., Haas, S., & Conway-Phillips, R. (2019). Optimizing strategies for care coordination and transition management: Recommendations for nursing education. *Nursing Economics, 37*(2), 77–85.

Zulman, D. (2019, July). *Care coordination for high-risk patients with multiple chronic conditions.* Retrieved from https://www.hsrd.research.va.gov/news/feature/care-coordination.cfm#1

6

Medication Adherence

Medication adherence is the act of taking medication as prescribed by a physician or licensed practitioner (Mospan, 2019). This means medicines are taken in the right dose, at the right time, for the indicated purpose and for the recommended period. According to *U. S. Pharmacist*, 50% of people do not take their medications as directed, which results in poor health outcomes, hospital admissions, increased health care costs, and decreased quality of life (Mospan, 2019). Nonadherence to a prescribed medication regimen results in increased medical resource utilization due to treatment failures and new medical problems caused by nonoptimal medication use (Aungst, 2018). These causal factors lead to downstream health service use and must be analyzed and included in any estimated costs for nonadherence (Aungst, 2018). The most often quoted figure as the cost for nonadherence is $300 billion annually; however, the *Annals of Internal Medicine* published new research that revealed the cost of drug-related morbidity and mortality resulting from nonoptimized medication therapy was $528.4 billion annually (Aungst, 2018). The researchers also showed that nearly 260,00 deaths could be attributed to nonoptimized medication therapy every year (Aungst, 2018). These are staggering data and can and should be used to encourage more aggressive medication management.

The reasons individuals are nonadherent can vary. They may be challenged with how to communicate the barriers that prevent adherence or unaware of the consequences of medication nonadherence (MNA); they do not understand the directions or instructions for taking medication; they are unable to pay for or afford the medication; or they may become confused about the dosing schedule, mistake one drug for another, do not feel any better after taking the medication, do not understand why they are taking the medication, or experience uncomfortable side effects.

"The Annals of Internal Medicine published new research that revealed the cost of drug-related morbidity and mortality resulting from nonoptimized medication therapy was $528.4 billion annually."

In 2013, the National Community Pharmacists Association (NCPA) published the first-ever Medication Adherence Report, an adherence report card for the United States. The report found that Americans with chronic conditions earned a C+ grade for medication adherence (National Community Pharmacists Association, 2013). The survey was conducted among Americans over 40 years of age who were taking prescribed medications for chronic conditions. The National Report Card on Adherence looked at medication-taking behaviors for 12 months (National Community Pharmacists Association, 2013):

- Failed to fill or refill a prescription
- Missed a dose
- Took lower or higher doses than prescribed
- Took old medication for a new problem
- Took someone else's medication
- Forgot whether they had taken medication

The study participants scored each of these elements on a scale of 0–10, with 0 equating to nonadherence in all behaviors and 10 equating to adherence in all behaviors (National Community Pharmacists Association, 2013). The average score was 79, or C+. Fifteen percent of the adults surveyed, or one in seven, were largely nonadherent with four or more of the behaviors listed (National Community Pharmacists Association, 2013).

The most common reasons for nonadherence are simply forgetting, running out of medication, being away from home, trying to save money, and experiencing side effects (National Community Pharmacists Association, 2013). The survey conducted by the NCPA also determined predictors of adherence. Here they are, in order of importance (National Community Pharmacists Association, 2013):

- A personal connection between a patient and pharmacist or pharmacy staff
- The affordability of medications

- Engagement in their health care
- The importance of taking medication
- The client/patient level of health understanding
- The severity of side effects (if any)

Understanding these predictors can assist providers and case managers in determining when nonadherence is a concern and address it in timely and proactive ways. These kinds of discussions strengthen personal connections with providers and improve communication.

Factors that contribute to adherence include adherence perceptions, health literacy, self-efficacy, cognitive abilities such as memory, coping, and problem-solving skills, and personal and cultural beliefs related to medication. Here are the factors in more detail (Shahin & Kennedy, 2019):

TABLE 6.1

Illness perception	Personal beliefs and expectations about illness
Personal beliefs about illness	Cognitive or emotional responses about the label of illness; the seriousness of the illness, the duration, and recovery; the consequences of a severe illness or disease; perceptions of what caused the illness; feelings that arise as a result of an illness, such as fear, anxiety, or depression
Spirituality and religiosity	The terms are often confused but are different. Spirituality is an individual's inner freedom to engage in faith and establish a relationship with a supreme being. Religiosity is the decision to follow prescribed beliefs, practices, and rituals that are centered around a supreme being.
Cultural beliefs	Culture and the resulting beliefs are a set of behavioral patterns, thoughts, manners, and actions shared by members of society; shared and passed on by succeeding generations
Self-management behaviors	These are impacted by health literacy and self-efficacy. Those with high health literacy have the social skills and motivation to access, understand, and use the information to maintain good health. Self-efficacy is the belief that one can manage any given situation or the ability to participate in self-care.

Creating an Atmosphere for Adherence

Patients/clients should never feel ashamed or afraid to ask questions about medications or other prescribed treatments. We, as clinicians, have the responsibility to create an environment that is safe and conducive to collaboration with our patients/clients. They should be able to ask any question without fear of shame or condescension.

An atmosphere for adherence will be dependent on the individual client/patient or population. For instance, seniors with cognitive impairment will require specialized interventions that would not be appropriate for other populations. For seniors with cognitive impairment, the level of impairment must first be assessed. A large segment of the American senior population is living independently with mild cognitive impairment. They may or may not have caregiver support or other support systems at home. These seniors are especially vulnerable to adverse events or illness from inappropriate medication use, which leads to hospital admissions or long-term care placement (Kroger et al., 2017).

Multiple strategies have been studied to improve medication adherence in seniors with mild cognitive impairment. These include simplifying medication regimens, using pill organizers, smart pill organizers, and dose-specific blister packs, and making telephone reminder calls. Unfortunately, there have been no studies that demonstrate one solution for adherence in the senior population. A significant contributor to poor adherence is the number of medications and frequency of dosing. Substantial evidence is available to demonstrate that if the prescribing physician and pharmacist work together to review the medications for any potential reduction, tapering or discontinuation might be possible without impacting health status and quality of life (Kroger et al., 2017). Deprescribing of medications may be the best strategy for vulnerable populations (Kroger et al., 2017).

Cost as a Determinant of Adherence

Chronic illness in the United States results in $1.3 trillion in direct health care costs and loss of productivity. Out-of-pocket costs can enable or impede access to care and services. Several studies have shown that lowering pharmacy copays has resulted in improved medication adherence (Abbass, Revere, & Mitchell, 2017). The association of the out-of-pocket costs burden is statistically significant for non-adherence. A $10 monthly increase in pharmacy copay results in a 7% higher likelihood of nonadherence (Abbass, Revere, & Mitchell, 2017). Neighborhood-related factors that impact adherence are households receiving public assistance: residents are 8% percent more likely to be nonadherent when compared to neighborhoods with fewer residents receiving public assistance (Abbass, Revere, & Mitchell, 2017). Other risk factors that impact adherence include the presence of comorbid conditions: for example, individuals with diabetes are 13% more likely to be nonadherent, and those with mental illness are 11% more likely to be nonadherent. The cost of multiple medications is a contributor to nonadherence in these situations.

The inability to afford medications is the most common cause of nonadherence but is not proactively addressed. Feasible strategies exist to assist clients/patients in reducing medication costs and can start with visits to their primary care providers (PCPs). Clients/patients may or may not be comfortable discussing affordability with their physicians but are more likely to share these types of concerns with nurses. When these concerns are not shared with physicians, cost-related nonadherence goes unrecognized (Carroll et al., 2019). A team-based approach to address adherence issues is a good strategy in the office setting to minimize competing demands on the physician (Carroll et al., 2019).

Medication reconciliation should take place at every office visit, ensuring that the medications reported as taken match with what has been ordered by the physician. This review is a perfect opportunity to ask the patient/client if the medications pose a financial burden. A nurse best conducts a Cost of Medication (COM) screening during "rooming" and nursing assessment and before the client/patient is seen by the provider. If clients/patients report financial barriers, the practice should have interventions at the ready:

> *"Deprescribing of medications may be the best strategy for vulnerable populations."*

- Familiarity with payer formularies to prevent prescribing of noncovered medications
- Have available discount coupons for select medications
- Make available $4 prescription plan information
- Recommend use of generics whenever possible

Supporting Adherence With Technology

The potential technology brings to adherence is exciting, but sometimes the technology supersedes the evidence. New applications for technology are created almost daily, but many are untested, and the evidence for clinical practice is incomplete. The challenge is that by the time research catches up to the technology, the technology has changed. More research is needed to establish large-scale applications that integrate eHealth, which includes electronic health information such as EHRs and associated databases, and mHealth, which includes mobile communication technology such as smartphones, tablets, applications, and Global Positioning System (GPS) activity trackers. There are numerous available and emerging technologies to assist with medication adherence. They range from low-tech solutions such as blister packs to high-tech reminder systems that generate phone calls and electronic reminders, innovative software applications that remind the individual to take medications, smart pill bottles, and sensors embedded in pills.

Examples of technological adherence tools include*:

- Abilify Mycite: ingestible event marker that tracks the taking of medication (https://www.abilifymycite.com/)
- ProAir Digihaler: stores usage data within inhaler and can be downloaded to an application for transmission to the provider (https://www.proairdigihaler.com)
- Prescription drug use-related software: software platforms that use digital health information to improve care. The development has been slow due to regulatory concerns. Still, the FDA is taking public comments for the development of a framework that will ensure the safety and efficacy of such tools and should encourage development. Examples include:
    - OncoPower: a platform that includes patient education and engagement, monitoring applications specific to prescription medications, and oncologist-to-oncologist consultation (https://oncopower.org/)
    - MediSafe: a free app that provides medication and refill reminders as well as drug interactions and allows families and caregivers to track adherence (http://medisafeapp.com)
    - MemoText: digital patient engagement platform that uses artificial intelligence to support medication adherence, access to a "nurse in the cloud," and support for individuals with schizophrenia (http://memotext.com)

**Mention of these adherence tools and devices is not to be interpreted as endorsement.*

Targets for future research include eHealth medical homes that use data from tracking devices and EHRs in an actionable report that can be sent to a provider to facilitate shared decision-making for treatment choices and supported adherence (Bender, 2018). The electronic medical home can facilitate information transfer among providers, health care institutions, and clients/patients to enable care coordination and better delivery. Examples include (Bender, 2018):

- Biosensors: smartphone connections and GPS-based functionality can be used to warn individuals of environmental hazards or other risks. Lifestyle biosensors such as Fitbit, Jawbone, and Lifetrak help individuals with diet, exercise, and sleep, and data can be integrated with an individual's personal EHR for even more personalized self-management.
- Incentives: technology can track and record adherent behaviors but also can automatically reward these behaviors with positive feedback or monetary credits toward copays.
- Big data: integration of mHealth and eHealth databases can reveal previously unrecognized patterns that can aid in risk stratification and develop more aggressive interventions.

Strategies to Improve Medication Adherence

The adherence strategies discussed earlier in this guide apply to all treatment, inclusive of medication. What is essential to understand about medication adherence, or the lack thereof, is that it may require multiple strategies. Some clients/patients may be nonadherent to medications resulting from psychological problems, some are willing to take medications but may be forgetful, some might be misinformed about the mechanisms of action, some may be concerned about adverse effects, some may have an absence of symptoms, and some may have poor follow-up, a lack of a trusted provider relationship, or difficulty affording the medication (Levenson, 2018). In this section, many strategies will be provided with resources included in the appendices.

The **Morisky Medication Adherence Scale (MMAS)** is a well-known and well-studied assessment tool used to assess medication adherence. It has received significant support since 2008 and has evolved from a single four-item scale to include an eight-item scale (Sison, 2018). The four-item scale evaluates forgetfulness and symptom severity, while the eight-item scale delves deeper into assessing feelings of pressure or reasons other than forgetfulness. The tool is easy to administer so as not to result in a burden to health care professionals and does not require a considerable time investment from the client/patient. Obtaining the information in real time allows for discussion at the point of care for feedback, teaching, coaching, support, encouragement, and coordination of interventions to overcome adherence barriers (see Appendix 12. The MMAS is protected by copyright. For permission to use the tool, visit http://www.moriskyscale.com/mmas-4--mmas-8-the-morisky-scales.html).

Tracking adherence can be achieved with client/patient self-reporting, monitoring claims data for pharmacy fills, and pill counts. Some of the newer technology can track adherence, but these are still not widely available and are costly. The American Medical Association, in partnership with the Society of General Internal Medicine, developed **STEPSforward**, a guide to medication adherence. Eight STEPS were identified to improve medication adherence (Brown, 2018). These steps and strategies are also detailed in Appendix 13.

1. Consider medication nonadherence first as a reason a patient's condition is not under control
2. Develop a process for routinely asking about medication adherence
3. Create a shame-and blame-free environment to discuss medications with the patient
4. Identify why the patient is not taking their medicine
5. Respond positively and thank the patient for sharing their behavior
6. Tailor the adherence solution to the individual patient
7. Involve the patient in developing their treatment plan
8. Set the patient up for success

"Medication adherence ... may require multiple strategies."

If the client/patient has a condition or conditions that are not well controlled, a review of what has been prescribed and their adherence must first be established before adding additional medications. If this step is not taken and more medications are added, a potentially dangerous situation could arise, especially if the client/patient decides to suddenly become adherent to both old and new medications. Regardless of the reason or reasons for nonadherence, it is vital to ask about medication-taking behavior in a nonjudgmental manner: "It must be difficult to take all of your pills. How often do you miss a dose?"

Developing a process for routinely asking about medication adherence can help with adherence challenges. Every encounter with a client/patient should include a review of their medications: "Are you still taking ________ (review each medication from the previous visit)?"

Be sure to ask if anything new has been added, by whom, and for what reason. To save on appointment time or other time constraints, a pre-visit/pre-encounter questionnaire can be developed that the client/patient completes related to medications. It should be specific to them based on their last appointment or encounter so the only checkboxes needed to be completed indicate if they are still taking the medication, if they ever miss a dose, and if so, how often. There can be a section for the client/patient to indicate any new medications. Medications can be reviewed by telephone prior to an appointment or encounter, or they can bring their medications to the appointment for review, also known as the "brown bag" medication review. Regardless of the process, this review of medications is a proactive measure to not only support adherence but also to get in front of nonadherence before more serious health issues arise. A worksheet to develop a medication review process can be found as Appendix 16.

Clients/patients may have legitimate reasons for not taking medications as prescribed; therefore, it is imperative that they feel comfortable enough to share this with the provider. Rather than confronting a client/patient by asking "Why aren't you taking your medicines?" the health care professional can, without blaming or shaming, say "Many people have trouble taking medicines on a regular basis. Is that something you have trouble with as well?" The client/patient is more likely to be honest about any difficulties experienced.

"Generic substitutions are often a useful and cost-effective strategy to improve adherence, but generic medicines almost always appear different than the name-brand drug. The client/patient will need to be made aware of the distinction so that no errors are made in medication taking."

Why someone does not take their medicines can be an intentional decision, and that decision may be made based on their personal experience, knowledge, or beliefs. Therefore, identifying why they are not taking prescribed medications is imperative to designing tailored interventions to improve adherence. Some clients/patients do not understand the progression of illness or that taking medication for an asymptomatic condition could prevent adverse outcomes. Clients/patients are often focused on short-term benefits and do not understand the implications of medication nonadherence on their future health.

There may be other reasons a client/patient is not taking their prescribed medications and they are not forthcoming with the causes because it could cause embarrassment. The client/patient may not have transportation to the pharmacy, or they may not be able to afford the medication or the copay. Clients/patients may stop taking medications when they begin to feel better or when symptoms subside. Again, education and support are required to help them understand the need to continue taking the medication long-term or until the provider tells them otherwise. Cost can be the primary reason clients/patients are nonadherent. A list of resources can be found in Appendix 10 that can be used to help your clients/patients access needed medications. Generic substitutions are often a useful and cost-effective strategy to improve adherence, but generic medicines almost always appear different than the name-brand drug. The client/patient will need to be made aware of the distinction so that no errors are made in medication taking. Nonadherence can also be unintentional: for example, when the client/patient forgets to take medications. For those who have difficulty remembering, help them define a routine activity that could be associated with medication taking, such as brushing teeth, drinking coffee, or making lunch. The medication could be physically placed in these areas, and the client/patient will remember to take them with the activity.

Working through the challenges with the client/patient means they have shared a great deal about themselves and their behaviors. As a result, we should make sure they know how much we appreciate being allowed into their world, and we should indeed consider this a privilege. Inadequate client/patient/provider communication can account for 55% of all nonadherence (Brown, 2018). As case managers, we should be supporting and encouraging the clients/patients to engage with their providers and ask questions so they can make decisions with their providers about their care and treatment.

Solutions to support adherence need to be tailored to the specific needs and preferences of the client/patient. Nonadherence, whether intentional or unintentional, can be resolved with custom-tailored interventions. For example, the client/patient who works the night shift might need medications that have longer half-lives or those that only require weekly or monthly dosing (Brown, 2018). Offer clients/patients options for convenience so medications are taken as prescribed; such options include convenient dosing, using a smartphone calendar or clock with alarms, utilizing a family member or other support person to help with reminders, and providing pill organizers, blister packs, alternative administration routes, and smart technology, such as applications that track adherence. For the elderly, especially those challenged with mild cognitive impairment, research demonstrates promising strategies, namely reducing the frequency of medication taking, educational strategies, and reminder techniques (Kroger et al., 2017). A recent approach showing significant promise is "deprescribing," which is the process by which a physician and pharmacist conduct a detailed medication review with the client/patient to determine their preferences, health status, and quality of life. Based on the shared decisions, tapering and even discontinuation of some medications can be implemented, and this intervention is demonstrating a reduction in overall polypharmacy in the elderly and reducing adverse medication events (Kroger et al., 2017).

Involving clients/patients in their treatment plans is likely to result in more engaged clients/patients. When providing new information, always do so only with permission, and find out what the client/patient knows and what they want to know before telling them what you think they should know. Allow time for questions, and provide information in small bites. Utilize the teach-back method, which can help determine how much the client/patient understands and how much information was absorbed. The best way to achieve teach-back is to impart knowledge to the client/patient and then ask them to deliver that information to another team member or a family member in your presence. If a client/patient remains reluctant to take a medication—whatever the reason—try to negotiate something that they might be willing to do to achieve the desired health outcome.

CASE STUDY

A client taking a beta-blocker for hypertension has not been consistently adherent because the medication makes him feel very fatigued. During an encounter, you note his blood pressure is 160/95. When you report this to the client/patient, he gets a concerned look on his face.

CM: "I see a concerned look on your face. Do you understand that this reading is high?"

> Pt: "Yes. I didn't think my blood pressure would be that high. I don't have a headache like I usually do when my blood pressure is up."
>
> CM: "So, you are now seeing that you do not always have symptoms when your blood pressure is elevated. Do you remember when we talked about that? Does this make you think any differently about taking medicine?"
>
> Pt: "What if I got more exercise and stopped eating salted food. Could I try that first?"
>
> CM: "This is certainly your decision, but I think we would need to run your idea by Dr. White first. Would you be willing to take your blood pressure at home every day and record it?"
>
> CM: "Would you be agreeable to 30 days if Dr. White signs off? And if there is no improvement in your blood pressure, will you agree to restart the beta-blocker?"

Success will be achieved when we make it easy for our clients/patients to adhere to their medication regimens. One of the most straightforward strategies is to make sure they have updated medication lists at every visit or encounter. Offer copies of the list to a family member or caregiver if the client/patient is agreeable or if the family member holds the health care proxy. Create an atmosphere of trust that is free of blame and shame. Make sure the client/patient feels they can contact you with any information and judgment will not be passed. Help them realize you are committed to understanding their struggles and experiences and will respect their preferences. Still, you will also keep them safe, and if you are ever concerned about safety, the appropriate action will be taken.

"We need our clients/patients to know we will support them with every available resource so they experience success."

If a client/patient is challenged with chronic illness, help them understand that they will likely need to take medication indefinitely; do not give them false or misleading information just to make them feel better. Help clients/patients understand that hospital admissions and ED visits are considered treatment failures and that with every hospital admission, their condition takes a step backward. We need our clients/patients to know we will support them with every available resource so they experience success.

Conclusion

Medication adherence is critical to patient health and safety. Improving medication adherence using the strategies provided in this guide will lead to the support of adherence in all aspects of an individual's health and well-being. What is most important for adherence to occur is the client/patient feels heard and their preferences are valued. Health care professionals should present themselves as the client's/patient's partner, not a parent or authority figure. Evidence-based practices can guide care but need to be tailored to the individual. It can be tempting to create a template for treating individuals with similar conditions, and while there are treatments that demonstrate success, not every client/patient will respond in the exact same manner.

The strategies and tools provided in this guide can be applied to any needed adherence behavior. Many tools and assessment examples have been included and can be found in the appendices. These resources can be taken to your place of practice, adapted to your population, and used to improve health outcomes. Case managers are best positioned to improve adherence because we are at the forefront of care coordination and care transitions. We interact with all members of the interdisciplinary team involved in a client's/patient's care and often are aware of challenges before other team members. The uniqueness of our role and function allows us to intervene before the client/patient experiences significant complication or harm.

Putting It Into Practice

Ask yourself these questions and reflect to target interventions for improving medication adherence:

- Case managers must fully appreciate the impact of poor medication adherence on health outcomes and health care costs. Have you examined your current caseload for evidence of poor adherence?
- If your patient/client is nonadherent with their prescription medications, do you know the *real* reason why?
- Do you know the predictors of nonadherence?
- Are you including the predictors in your assessments?
  Case managers must help create and support a safe and collaborative environment for their patients/clients.
- Do you know how much your patients/clients pay for their prescriptions?

(Continued)

Putting It Into Practice (*Continued*)

- Do you have resources ready to help patients/clients obtain and pay for their prescriptions?
- Adherence is being supported by technology—make yourself familiar with what may be available to help your patients/clients. Are any of them using technology?
- Do you use tools and scales to assess for adherence and adherence behaviors? For example, MMAS.
- How are you tracking adherence? Consider using technology to track adherence but involve and engage the patient/client in adherence: STEPSforward
- Every patient/client is different—How will you develop personalized strategies for each individual?
- Have you thought about how to create an atmosphere that is blame-free and geared for success?

References

Abbass, I., Revere, L., & Mitchell, J. (2017). Medication nonadherence: The role of cost, community, and individual factors. *Health Services Research, 52*(4), 1511–1533. doi:10.1111/1475-6773.12547

Aungst, T. (2018, June 1). *Does nonadherence really cost the health care system $300 billion annually?* Pharmacy Times. https://www.pharmacytimes.com/contributor/timothy-aungst-pharmd/2018/06/does-nonadherence-really-cost-the-health-care-system-300-billion-annually

Bender, B. (2018). Technology interventions for nonadherence: A new approach to an old problem. *Journal of Allergy and Clinical Immunology, 6*(3), 794–800. doi:https://doi.org/10.1016/j.jaip.2017.10.029

Brown, M. (2018). Medication adherence: Improve patient outcomes and reduce costs. *AMA STEPSforward.* American Medical Association. https://edhub.ama-assn.org/

Carroll, J., Farah, S., Fortuna, R., Lanigan, A., Sanders, M., & Venci, J. (2019). Addressing medication costs during primary care visits: A before–after study of team-based training. *Annals of Internal Medicine, 170*, S46–S53. doi:10.7326/M18-2011

Kroger, E., Tatar, O., Vedel, I., Gigue`re, A., Voyer, P., Guillaumie, L., & Gre´goire, J. (2017). Improving medication adherence among community-dwelling seniors with cognitive impairment: A systematic review of interventions. *International Journal of Clinical Pharmacy, 39,* 641–656. doi:10.1007/s11096-017-0487-6

Levenson, J. (2018). Psychological factors affecting other medical conditions: Management. *UpToDate.*

Mospan, C. (2019, June 18). *Patient counseling approaches to enhance medication adherence.* U.S. Pharmacist. https://www.uspharmacist.com/article/patient-counseling-approaches-to-enhance-medication-adherence

National Community Pharmacists Association. (2013). *Medication adherence in America: A national report.* Alexandria, VA: NCPA.

Neiman, A., Ruppar, T., Ho, M., Garber, L., Weidle, P., Hong, Y., & George, M. (2017, November 17). CDC grand rounds: Improving medication adherence for chronic disease management — innovations and opportunities. *Morbidity and Mortality Weekly Report, 66*(45), 1248–1251.

Shahin, W., & Kennedy, G. A. (2019). The impact of personal and cultural beliefs on medication adherence of patients with chronic illnesses: a systematic review. *Patient Preference and Adherence, 13,* 1019–1035.

Sison, G. (2018, December 9). *The Morisky Medication Adherence Scale: An overview.* Pillsy. https://www.pillsy.com/articles/the-morisky-medication-adherence-scale-definition-alternatives-and-overview

APPENDICES: TABLE OF CONTENTS

APPENDIX 1

PRAPARE

Protocol for Responding to and Assessing Patients' Assets, Risks, and Experiences

PRAPARE

Protocol for Responding to and Assessing Patients' Assets, Risks, and Experiences

Source: http://www.nachc.org/research-and-data/prapare/toolkit/.

Tool kit available to assist in gathering data to better understand social determinants of health to meet the needs of clients/patients.

PRARARE is an evidence-based and stakeholder-driven method for assessing and collecting data related to the social determinants of health. The full resource is available at:

https://www.nachc.org/research-and-data/prapare/toolkit/

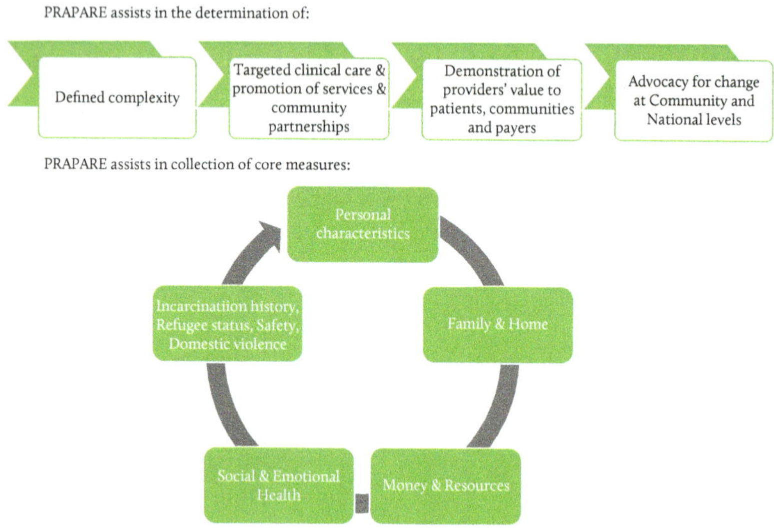

FIGURE A.1.1

Source: https://www.nachc.org/wp-content/uploads/2020/07/NACHC_PRAPARE_ALL-Updated-7.13.20-Translations-Included.pdf

APPENDIX 2

Health-Related and Quality of Life Scales

ProQOL 5

https://proqol.org/ProQol_Test.html

The ProQOL 5 is available free and does not require permission, providing the scale is not changed and the author is cited. The scale is available in 26 languages, but specific translations can be requested on the website.

Professional Quality of Life Scale (ProQOL)

Compassion Satisfaction and Compassion Fatigue (ProQOL) Version 5 (2009) For Caregivers

When you *[help]* people you have direct contact with their lives. As you may have found, your compassion for those you *[help]* can affect you in positive and negative ways. Below are some questions about your experiences, both positive and negative, as a *[helper]*. Consider each of the following questions about you and your current work situation. Select the number that honestly reflects how frequently you experienced these things in the last 30 days.

1=Never 2=Rarely 3=Sometimes 4=Often 5=Very Often

_____ 1. I am happy.
_____ 2. I am preoccupied with more than one person I *[help]*.
_____ 3. I get satisfaction from being able to *[help]* people.
_____ 4. I feel connected to others.
_____ 5. I jump or am startled by unexpected sounds.
_____ 6. I feel invigorated after working with those I *[help]*.
_____ 7. I find it difficult to separate my personal life from my life as a *[helper]*.
_____ 8. I am not as productive at work because I am losing sleep over traumatic experiences of a person I *[help]*.
_____ 9. I think that I might have been affected by the traumatic stress of those I *[help]*.
_____ 10. I feel trapped by my job as a *[helper]*.
_____ 11. Because of my *[helping]*, I have felt "on edge" about various things.
_____ 12. I like my work as a *[helper]*.
_____ 13. I feel depressed because of the traumatic experiences of the people I *[help]*.
_____ 14. I feel as though I am experiencing the trauma of someone I have *[helped]*.
_____ 15. I have beliefs that sustain me.
_____ 16. I am pleased with how I am able to keep up with *[helping]* techniques and protocols.
_____ 17. I am the person I always wanted to be.
_____ 18. My work makes me feel satisfied.
_____ 19. I feel worn out because of my work as a *[helper]*.
_____ 20. I have happy thoughts and feelings about those I *[help]* and how I could help them.
_____ 21. I feel overwhelmed because my case [work] load seems endless.
_____ 22. I believe I can make a difference through my work.
_____ 23. I avoid certain activities or situations because they remind me of frightening experiences of the people I *[help]*.
_____ 24. I am proud of what I can do to *[help]*.
_____ 25. As a result of my *[helping]*, I have intrusive, frightening thoughts.
_____ 26. I feel "bogged down" by the system.
_____ 27. I have thoughts that I am a "success" as a *[helper]*.
_____ 28. I can't recall important parts of my work with trauma victims.
_____ 29. I am a very caring person.
_____ 30. I am happy that I chose to do this work.

B. Hudnall Stamm, "Professional Quality of Life Scale (ProQOL)," Professional Quality of Life: Compassion Satisfaction and Fatigue Version 5 (ProQOL).

Nottingham Health Profile (NHP)

Subjective measure of an individual's health status typically performed in the primary care setting. The tool has been translated into 24 languages and is copyrighted by Galen Research. Galen Research is a group of scientists dedicated to developing and measuring patient-reported outcomes. You can view a sample of the NHP and get information on licensing at www.galen-research.com/contact

EuroQol (EQ) (EQ-5D)

EQ is a family of instruments that can be used in clinical trials as well as in clinical settings. The EQ-5D evaluates five dimensions: mobility, self-care, usual activities, pain/discomfort, and anxiety/depression. Commercial use requires licensing; nonprofits may use at no cost after registration. To inquire: https://www.euroqol.org

36-Item Short Form Survey (SF-36)

Generic tool developed to evaluate patient-reported quality of life measures. The survey is widely accepted by Medicare and managed care organizations. No licensing or permissions are required for use. For more information: https://www.rand.org/health-care/surveys_tools/mos/36-item-short-form.html

WHO-5 Well-Being Scale (WHO-5)

A survey developed by the Psykiatrisk Centre in North Zealand, Denmark for the World Health Organization. The five-item survey evaluates mood and, to some extent, motivation. To view the tool: https://www.psykiatri-regionh.dk/who-5/Pages/default.aspx

The tool is copyrighted. For permission contact:

Psykiatrisk Centre North Zealand
Psykiatrisk Research Unit
Dyrehavevej 48
DK-3400 Hillerød
+45 3864 3000

APPENDIX 3

Accountable Health Communities Health-Related Social Needs Screening Tool

https://innovation.cms.gov/Files/worksheets/ahcm-screeningtool.pdf

The Center for Medicare and Medicaid Innovation has made available this tool that assesses the needs in the five core domains that can be alleviated by community services. The five domains include housing, transportation, food, utilities, and interpersonal safety. Screening for social needs has not been standardized to date, but CMMI is recommending use of the tool for all Accountable Health Communities, and it has been reviewed by the National Academy of Medicine.

The 10-question survey is meant for the individual to answer, but a parent or caregiver can also complete it. Multiple-choice answers are available for selection, and any answer that is underlined may indicate vulnerability. Here is an example:

Living Situation

1. What is your living situation today?

- I have a steady place to live
- I have a place to live today, but I am worried about losing it in the future
- I do not have a steady place to live (I am temporarily staying with others, in a hotel, in a shelter, living outside on the street, on a beach, in a car, abandoned building, bus or train station, or in a park)

Supplemental questions are available to screen for vulnerability in finance, education, family and community support, physical activity, substance use, mental health, and disabilities.

APPENDIX 4

Patient Activation Measure

The tool can assist in predicting ED use, admissions, and adherence. Licensing and cost information can be accessed at: https://www.insigniahealth.com/products/pam-survey. The PAM has been studied for over 15 years and produced more than 500 studies demonstrating validity. This is an example of a completed study from 2004.

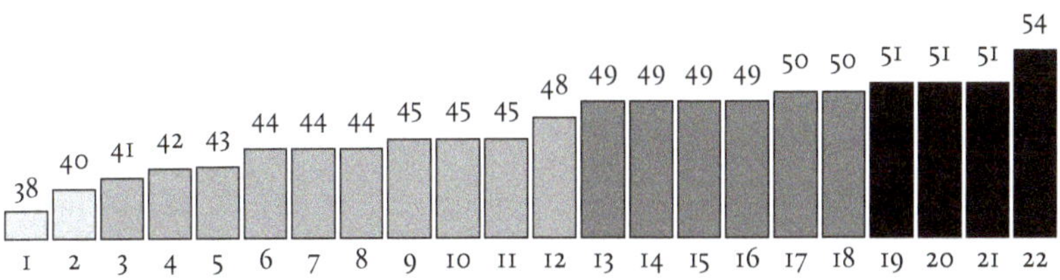

	Believes Active Role Important	SEM	Infit	Outfit
1	When all is said and done, I am the person who is responsible for managing my health condition	0.39	0.92	0.88
2	Taking an active role in my own health care is the most important factor in determining my health and ability to function	0.39	1.08	1.06
	Confidence and Knowledge to Take Action	**SEM**	**Infit**	**Outfit**
3	I know what each of my prescribed medications do	0.44	1.02	0.99
4	I am confident I can tell my health care provider concerns I have even when he or she does not ask	0.39	0.86	0.82
5	I am confident that I can tell when I need to go get medical care and when I can handle a health problem myself	0.39	0.71	0.67

(Continued)

	Confidence and Knowledge to Take Action	SEM	Infit	Outfit
6	I know the lifestyle changes like diet and exercise that are recommended for my health condition	0.39	0.92	0.94
7	I am confident that I can follow through on medical treatment I need to do at home	0.39	0.91	0.86
8	I am confident that I can take actions that will help prevent or minimize some symptoms or problems associated with my health condition	0.39	0.85	0.81
9	I am confident that I can find trustworthy sources of information about my health condition and my health choices	0.38	0.85	0.81
10	I am confident that I can follow through on medical recommendations my heath care provider makes, such as changing my diet or doing regular exercise	0.38	0.92	0.88
11	Understand the nature and causes of my health condition(s)	0.40	0.95	0.91
12	I know the different medical treatment options for my health condition	0.39	0.84	0.80
	Taking Action	**SEM**	**Infit**	**Outfit**
13	I have been able to maintain the lifestyle changes for my health that I have made	0.37	0.91	0.90
14	I know how to prevent further problems with my health condition	0.36	0.95	0.92
15	I know about the self-treatments for my health condition	0.37	0.87	0.85
16	I have made the changes in my lifestyle like diet exercise that are recommended for my health condition	0.37	1.30	1.34
17	I am confident I can figure out solutions when new situations or problems arise with my health condition	0.36	1.00	1.02
18	I am able to handle symptoms of my health condition on my own at home	0.36	1.13	1.15

(Continued)

Staying the Course under Stress		SEM	Infit	Outfit
19	I am confident that I can maintain lifestyle changes like diet and exercise even during times of stress	0.35	0.90	0.91
20	I am able to handle problems of my health condition on my own at home	0.35	1.07	1.13
21	I am confident I can keep my health problems from interfering with the things I want to do	0.35	1.16	1.25
22	Maintaining the lifestyle changes that are recommended for my health condition is too hard to do on daily basis	0.33	1.44	1.64

Judith H Hibbard, Jean Stockard, Eldon R Mahoney, and Martin Tusler, "Figure 2: Final Patient Activation Measure (PAM) with Item Calibrations, from 'Development of the Patient Activation Measure (PAM): Conceptualizing and Measuring Activation in Patients and Consumers,'" *Health Services Research*, vol. 39, no. 4, pp. 1017.

Shared Decision-Making

In support of the shared decision-making framework included in this guide, the Agency for Healthcare Research and Quality (AHRQ) provides additional resources to assist in creating an environment for clinicians and clients/patients to collaborate in care. AHRQ makes available SHARE to provide health care professionals with the training and tools needed to implement shared decision-making.

The SHARE Approach: A Model for Shared Decision-Making:

https://www.ahrq.gov/sites/default/files/publications/files/share-approach_factsheet.pdf

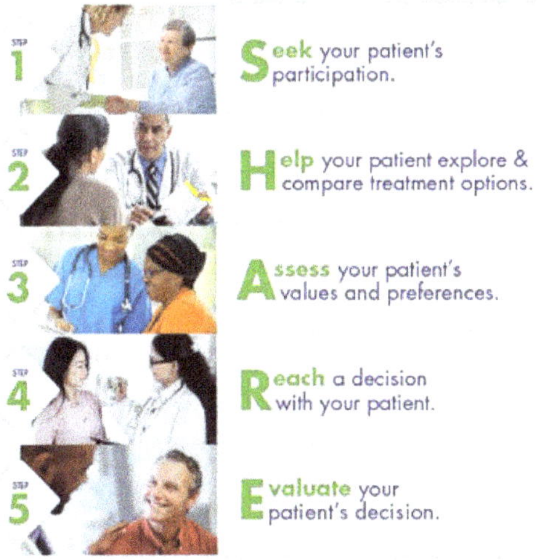

FIGURE A.5.1

Source: https://www.ahrq.gov/health-literacy/professional-training/shared-decision/tools/factsheet.html.

The SHARE Approach: A Model for Shared Decision-Making—Fact Sheet. Content last reviewed September 2016. Agency for Healthcare Research and Quality. Rockville, MD. https://bit.ly/2QAytcO

APPENDIX 6

Emotional Intelligence

Emotional intelligence (EI) is the ability to identify and manage one's own emotions as well as the emotions of others.

To possess EI, three skills are needed (*Psychology Today*, 2020):

1. The ability to identify and name one's own emotions
2. The ability to harness emotions and apply them to thinking and problem-solving
3. The ability to manage or regulate emotions when necessary and help others do the same

An individual who is emotionally intelligent is highly conscious of both positive and negative feelings: frustration, sadness, or even more subtle emotions. Some individuals are tuned into the emotions of others and/or sensitive to emotional signals. These individuals make better friends, leaders, and parents. The good news is these skills can be honed. Emotional intelligence (EI) is also known as emotional quotient (EQ).

The following are the Five Categories of Emotional Intelligence (Bressert, 2016):

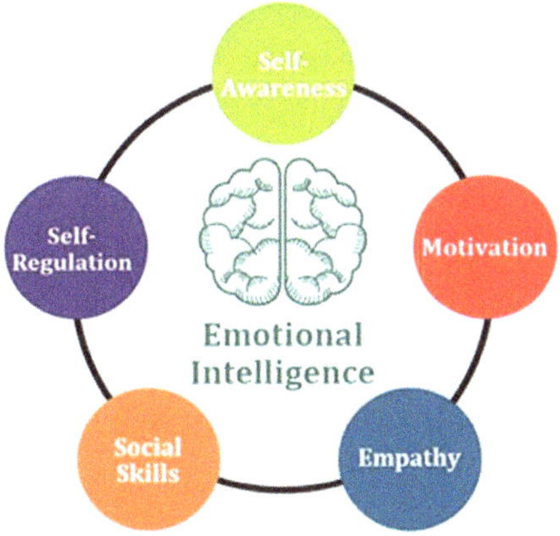

FIGURE A.6.1 Five Categories of Emotional Intelligence.

The Five Categories of Emotional Intelligence	
Self-awareness	To recognize an emotion as it happens; recognize emotions and their effects; having the confidence in your own self-worth and capabilities
Self-regulation	One may have little control over when emotions occur but has control over how long emotions have an impact; able to recast a situation in a positive light through a positive activity like walking, meditating, prayer; has self-control, is trustworthy and conscientious, and can adapt through innovation
Motivation	Having goals and a positive attitude; positivity occurs with practice, the ability to stop negative thoughts as they occur, having the drive to achieve; having initiative and optimism
Empathy	How others feel is important; willing to learn how to recognize the emotions of others; being service oriented; understanding the emotions of others
Social skills	Having positive interpersonal skills, influence; ability to communicate; leadership qualities; change catalyst; able to manage conflict; build bonds and collaborative teams

Testing and training in emotional intelligence are available from reputable sources like *Psychology Today* and PsychCentral.

https://www.psychologytoday.com/us/basics/emotional-intelligence

https://psychcentral.com/blog/the-benefits-of-emotional-intelligence/

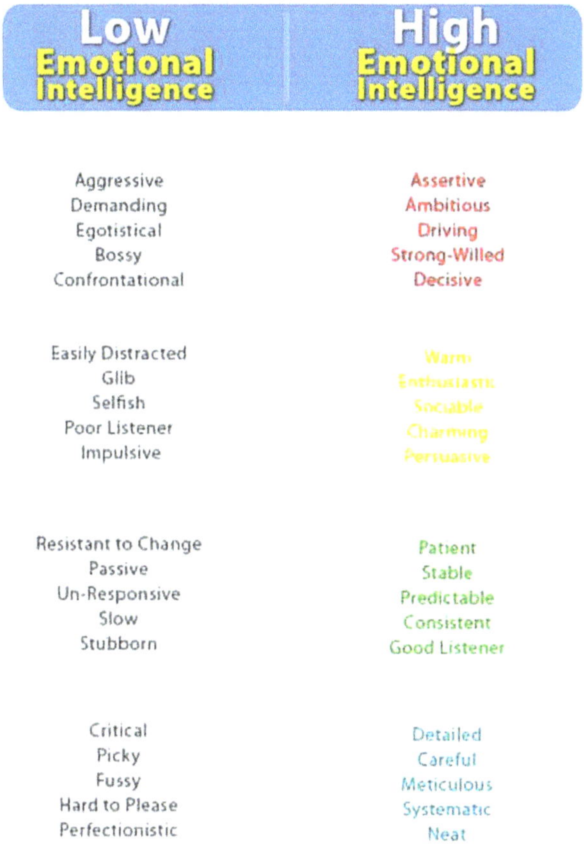

FIGURE A.6.2 Low vs. High Emotional Intelligence.

Source: https://positivepsychology.com/emotional-intelligence-frameworks/.

APPENDIX 7

Motivational Interviewing

Motivational interviewing (MI) is a well-validated communication method that addresses an individual's ambivalence about the need to make changes—it is a discussion about change. It is a patient-centered method originally developed to promote health among excessive drinkers and then with tobacco users. When applied as a patient-centered approach, rapport must be established and then an agenda set for what is to be accomplished. The following is but a brief synopsis of the MI method. Training is strongly recommended.

Questions to ask:

- What would you like to talk about?
- What would you like to be different?
- How do you think we make things different?

MI is not a method one can learn from a 2-hour presentation. It is a method that requires investment in learning, time, and practice. There are many factors that impact the clinician's ability to begin discussing change with a client/patient. Building rapport has been mentioned, but it also includes understanding the spirit in which MI is practiced.

The Four Elements of MI

- Acceptance
    - Absolute worth: valuing the inherent worth of every human being
    - Accurate empathy: demonstrating genuine interest in an individual and making every effort to understand their perspective

    - Affirmation: acknowledge the strengths an individual has rather than telling them what is wrong and how to fix it
- Compassion
    - The promotion of an individual's welfare and giving priority to their needs; a desire to relieve their suffering
- Evocation
    - Helping an individual identify and call forth strengths that can help them make changes
- Partnership
    - Someone leads and someone follows, but when it is a good partnership, no one knows which one

Communication Style

MI is conducted using a guiding style of communication that at times may be directive but at others follows the individual's lead

Communication Techniques

- Open-ended questions
    - Asked in a way that more conversation ensues
- Affirmations
    - Acknowledge an individual's successes
- Reflective listening
    - Convey to the individual what you heard to ensure understanding
- Summarizing
    - Repeating back a summary of the conversation to avoid misunderstanding and to plan what happens next

Signs of Readiness to Change and How to Support

High-level readiness:

"I am ready to do this!"
"I feel really good about ________."
How you support: "So what will you do next?"

Low-level readiness:

"I guess I could try."
"I'm not so sure. ... I guess I could give a try."
How you encourage: "What might help you feel more confident?"

Resources for Motivational Interviewing

Motivational Interviewing for Health Care Professionals: A Sensible Approach. 2nd Edition.

Bruce A. Berger; William A. Villaume

Health Behavior Change: A Guide For Practitioners.

Stephen Rollnick, Pip Mason, Chris Butler

APPENDIX 8

LACE Tool

LACE Index Scoring Tool for Risk Assessment of Hospital Readmission

Step 1. Length of Stay

Length of stay (including day of admission and discharge): ________ days

Length of stay (days)	Score (circle as appropriate)
1	1
2	2
3	3
4–6	4
7–13	5
14 or more	7

→ **L**

Step 2. Acuity of Admission

Was the patient admitted to hospital via the emergency department? If yes, enter 3 in Box A. Otherwise, enter 0 in Box A.

A

Step 3. Comorbidities

C

Condition (definitions and notes on reverse)	Score (circle as appropriate)	
Previous myocardial infarction	+1	If the TOTAL score is between 0 and 3, enter the score into Box C. If the score is 4 or higher, enter 5 into Box C.
Cerebrovascular disease	+1	
Peripheral vascular disease	+1	
Diabetes without compli-cations	+1	
Congestive heart failure	+2	
Diabetes with end organ damage	+2	
Chronic pulmonary disease	+2	
Mild liver or renal disease	+2	
Any tumor (including lymphoma or leukemia)	+2	
Dementia	+3	
Connective tissue disease	+3	
AIDS	+4	
Moderate or severe liver or renal disease	+4	
Metastatic solid tumor	+6	
TOTAL		

Step 4. Emergency department visits

E

How many times has the patient visited an emergency department in the 6 months prior to admission (not including the emergency department visit immediately preceding the current admission)?

Enter this number or 4 (whichever is smaller) in Box E.

Add the numbers in Box L, Box A, Box C, and Box E to generate the LACE score and enter into the box below.

LACE

LACE SCORE Risk of Readmission: ≥ 10 High Risk

Condition	Definition and/or notes
Previous myocardial infarction	Any previous definite or probable myocardial infarction
Cerebrovascular disease	Any previous stroke or transient ischemic attack (TIA)
Peripheral vascular disease	Intermittent claudication, previous surgery or stenting, gangrene or acute ischemia, untreated abdominal or thoracic aortic aneurysm
Diabetes without micro-vascular complications	No retinopathy, nephropathy, or neuropathy
Congestive heart failure	Any patient with symptomatic CHF whose symptoms have responded to appropriate medications
Diabetes with end organ damage	Diabetes with retinopathy, nephropathy, or neuropathy
Chronic pulmonary disease	Stage III or higher COPD or other chronic lung condition
Mild liver or renal disease	Cirrhosis but no portal hypertension (i.e., no varices, no ascites) or chronic hepatitis Chronic renal disease, ESRD
Any tumor (including lymphoma or leukemia)	Solid tumors must have been treated within the last 5 years; includes chronic lymphocytic leukemia (CLL) and polycythemia vera (PV)
Dementia	Any cognitive deficit?
Connective tissue disease	Systemic lupus erythematosus (SLE), polymyositis, mixed connective tissue disease, moderate to severe rheumatoid arthritis, and polymyalgia rheumatica
AIDS	AIDS-defining opportunistic infection or CD4 < 200
Moderate or severe liver or renal disease	Cirrhosis with portal hypertension (e.g., ascites or variceal bleeding) End-stage renal disease, hemodialysis, or peritoneal dialysis
Metastatic solid tumor	Any metastatic tumor

LACE SCORE Grid

Item	Description	Score
L	Length of Stay	
A	Acuity of Admission	
C	Comorbidities	
E	Emergency Department Visits	
Total Score	If ≥10, High Readmission Risk	

APPENDIX 9

"Ask Me Three"

Available through the Institute for Healthcare Improvement and provides resources for patient education in multiple languages. IHI provides, through a nonexclusive, nontransferable license, certain Ask Me 3 materials and resources for download and distribution free of charge to aid in the promotion of health communication, including health literacy and increased patient safety.

http://www.ihi.org/resources/Pages/Tools/Ask-Me-3-Good-Questions-for-Your-Good-Health.aspx

APPENDIX 10

Rapid Estimate of Adult Literacy in Medicine—Short Form (REALM-SF)

REALM-SF Score Sheet

Patient ID #: _____ Date: ________ Examiner Initials: ________

Behavior	________
Exercise	________
Menopause	________
Rectal	________
Antibiotics	________
Anemia	________
Jaundice	________
TOTAL SCORE	________

Administering the REALM-SF:

Suggested Introduction:

"Providers often use words that patients don't understand. We are looking at words providers often use with their patients in order to improve communication between health care providers and patients. Here is a list of medical words.

Starting at the top of the list, please read each word aloud to me. If you don't recognize a word, you can say 'pass' and move on to the next word."

Interviewer: Give the participant the word list. If the participant takes more than 5 seconds on a words, say "pass" and point to the next word. Hold this scoring sheet so that it is not visible to the participant.

Source: https://www.ahrq.gov/health-literacy/research/tools/index.html#rapid.

APPENDIX 11

Financial Resources for Access to Medications and Medication Assistance

Rx Assist www.rxassist.org

Directory of patient assistance programs; a database is available to search by drug name; RxVantage is a network to search for drug reps in your area to help with access to medication coupons and samples

NeedyMeds www.needymeds.com

- Drug discount card
- Drug pricing calculator
- Subscribe to alerts for patient assistance programs
- Subscribe to alerts for programs related to specific diseases
- Healthfinder: a medical crowd-funding foundation providing financial assistance for medical expenses through private donations

Medication Assist Tool https://medicineassistancetool.org (www.pparx.org)

Search engine for patients looking for medication assistance

Rx Hope https://www.rxhope.com

Online search by drug name for resources. Health care professionals can submit applications for patients.

Center for Benefits https://www.ncoa.org/professionals/benefits/center-for-benefits-access

Division of the National Council on Aging assisting seniors and young adults with disabilities in paying for Medicare Part D coverage, accessing unaffordable prescription drugs and state pharmaceutical assistance programs (SPAPs)

Rx Outreach https://rxoutreach.org/health-care-professionals

Health care professionals can search medication access for the uninsured

GoodRx: https://www.goodrx.com/how-goodrx-works

Provides discounts for medications, some as low as $4 per prescription, regardless of insured status. A GoodRx Card can be obtained by searching by drug name.

APPENDIX 12

Morisky Medication Adherence Scale (MMAS)

The MMAS is a validated diagnostic tool to assess medication adherence. The scale is available as either four-item or eight-item assessments. The assessment is protected by copyright law, and licensing must be obtained before use. You must contact Dr. Donald Morisky and request permission at: http://www.moriskyscale.com/mmas-4-mmas-8-the-morisky-scales.html

You indicated that you are taking medication for your (identify health concern, such as "high blood pressure"). Individuals have identified several issues regarding their medication-taking behavior and we are interested in your experiences. There is no right or wrong answer. Please answer each question based on your personal experience with your [health concern] medication. Interviewers may self identify regarding difficulties they may experience concerning medication-taking behavior.		
(Please circle the correct number)		
	No=0	**Yes=1**
1. Do you sometimes forget to take your [health concern] pills?		
2. People sometimes miss taking their medications for reasons other than forgetting. Thinking over the past two weeks, were there any days when you did not take your [health concern] medicine?		
3. Have you ever cut back or stopped taking your medication without telling your doctor, because you felt worse when you took it?		
4. When you travel or leave home, do you sometimes forget to bring along your [health concern] medication?		
5. Did you take your [health concern] medicine yesterday?		

(Continued)

(Please circle the correct number)		
	No=0	Yes=1
6. When you feel like your [health concern] is under control, do you sometimes stop taking your medicine?		
7. Taking medication everyday is a real inconvenience for some people. Do you ever feel hassled about sticking to your blood pressure treatment plan?		
8. How often do you have difficulty remembering to take all your medications? (**Please circle the correct number**) Never/Rarely........**0** Once in a while........**1** Sometimes........**2** Usually........**3** All the time........**4**		

Source: Donald E. Morisky, Alfonso Ang, Marie Krousel-Wood, and Harry J. Ward, "Fig. 1. MAQ (Medication Adherence Questionnaire), from 'Predictive Validity of a Medication Adherence Measure for Hypertension Control,'" *Journal of Clinical Hypertension*, vol. 10, no. 5. Copyright © 2008 by John Wiley & Sons, Inc.

For additional information, contact: Donald E. Morisky, Sc.D., M.S.P.H., Sc.M., e-mail: dmorisky@ucla.edu; phone: (310) 825-8508

APPENDIX 13

STEPSforward

Consider Medication nonadherence first as a reason for a patient's uncontrolled health condition(s).	Review what has been prescribed and the rate of adherence. Do not add or remove medications until this has been established.
Develop a process for routinely asking about medication adherence.	Inquire about medications at every encounter: "Let's take a few minutes to review your medicines. Are you still taking ___? Are you taking any new medicines? Have you stopped taking any medicine?" Inquire about any adverse effects. To save time during office visits, develop a brief questionnaire tailored to the patient that can be completed before appointments, reviewing medicines, side effects, and any changes. Medication reviews can also be conducted by telephone before appointments.
Create a shame- and blame-free environment to discuss medications.	"It must be difficult sometimes to take medicines. How often do you miss a dose?"
Identify why the patient is not taking medicines.	If doses are missed, ask the reason without judgment: "How do you feel after taking ____?" "What is your understanding of why this medicine has been ordered?" "Do you believe the medicine will help you?" "I know this medicine can be expensive. Is this a problem for you?"

(Continued)

Respond positively and thank them for sharing their behavior.	"It can sometimes be difficult to talk about why we do or don't choose to take medicines. Please know I appreciate what you have told me because I understand better how to help you."
Tailor the adherence solution to the individual.	Once the reason for nonadherence is determined, develop recommended solutions.
Involve the patient in developing the treatment plan.	Propose recommended solutions to the patient for their approval and consent (e.g., generics, dosing, patient assistance programs). Negotiate their willingness to adhere.
Set the patient up for success.	Make available every tool and intervention that could lead to successful adherence. Make the patient aware of your availability for support and for alterations to treatment if needed.

APPENDIX 14

Ten Principles of Patient-Centered Care

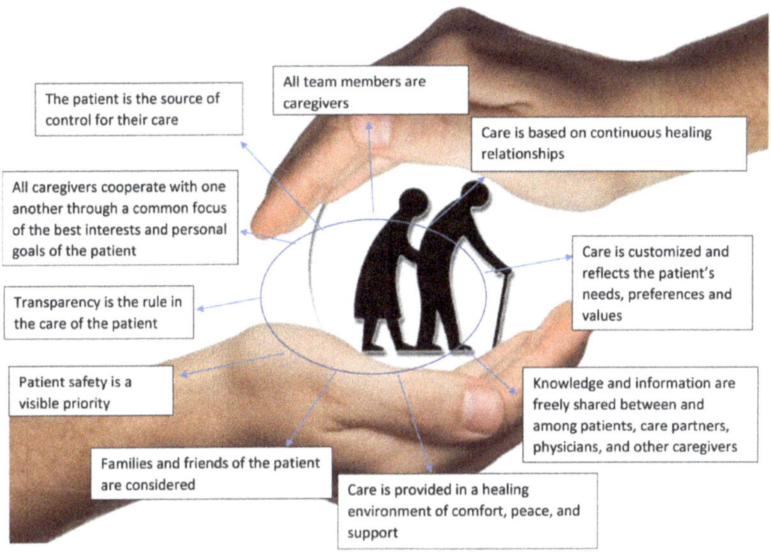

FIGURE A.14.1 Ten Principles of Patient-Centered Care.

Source: https://pixabay.com/illustrations/seniors-care-for-the-elderly-1505935/

APPENDIX 15

Care Transition Worksheet

This worksheet can be used to develop and customize your own process for transitions of care. It is best to work with an interdisciplinary team to gather all the needed information and then to coordinate needed care and services using resources for which each discipline is aware. The post-discharge follow-up can guide the case manager following the client/patient after discharge.

Discharge Planning	
Determine Readmission Risk	**Use the LACE tool or other risk assessment** -facilitate additional supports for better disease/condition control (e.g., home health, telehealth)
Assess Vulnerabilities	**Ability to attend appointments** -need to coordinate transportation **Presence of social support** -coordinate community resources if available **Presence of financial challenges** -coordinate assistance with rent, utilities, food **Safe environment** -facilitate safe housing if needed **Facilitate interventions for abuse if needed**
Ability to Obtain Medication	**Can pick up from pharmacy** **Mail order** **Needs assistance with copay** -pharmacy assistance programs **Needs assistance with obtaining medication due to cost** -pharmacy assistance programs

(Continued)

Discharge Planning	
Independent with ADLs/IADLs	**Needs assistive equipment** - equipment for delivery before discharge -coordinate nonclinical supports if available

Post-Discharge Follow-Up		
Post-Discharge Appointment Complete	Yes	No
Review Medications/Medication Adherence	Yes	No
Changes in Medication	Yes	No
Changes in Condition		
Next Scheduled Appointment		
Are All Needs Met?	Yes	No
If All Needs Are Not Met, What Is Needed?		

APPENDIX 16

Medication Adherence Worksheet

This worksheet can be used to develop a customized process for determining your client/patient adherence. The process can be developed for client/patient self-completion or one that is completed by interview.

In the box to the right, please list each of the medicines you take and why your doctor prescribed them.		
Have you stopped taking any medicines since your last appointment?	Yes	No
If yes, please list them and the reason for stopping		
Have you started any new medicines since your last appointment?	Yes	No
If yes, please list them and provide the name of the doctor who prescribed and the reason		
Do you ever miss taking any of your medicines?	Yes	No
If yes, please list which ones		
How often do miss a dose?		
Do your medicines cause any side effects?	Yes	No
If yes, please describe the side effects		
Do you have difficulty paying for any of your medicines?	Yes	No
Is there any other reason that you might not want to take your medicines?		

APPENDIX 17

Telehealth Resources

Medicare Telehealth Tool Kit

Medicare Coverage information of virtual services

https://www.cms.gov/newsroom/fact-sheets/medicare-telemedicine-health-care-provider-fact-sheet

Type of Service	What is the Service?	HCPCS/CPT Code	Patient Relationship with Provider
Medicare Telehealth Visits	A visit with a provider that uses telecommunication systems between a provider and a patient	Common telehealth services include: 99201–99215 (office or other outpatient visits) G0425–G0427 (telehealth consultations, emergency department, or initial inpatient) G0406–G0408 (follow-up inpatient telehealth consultations furnished to beneficiaries in hospitals or SNFs) For a complete list: https://www.cms.gov/Medicare/Medicare-General-Information/Telehealth/Telehealth-Codes	For new* or established patients. *To the extent the 1135 waiver requires an established relationship, HHS will not conduct audits to ensure that such a prior relationship existed for claims submitted during this public health emergency.

(Continued)

Virtual Check-In	A brief (5–10 minutes) check-in with your practitioner via telephone or other telecommunications device to decide whether an office visit or other service is needed. A remote evaluation of recorded video and/or images submitted by an established patient.	HCPCS code G2012 HCPCS code G2010	For established patients
E-Visits	A communication between a patient and their provider through an online patient portal.	99421 99422 99423 G2061 G2062 G2063	For established patients.

Source: https://www.cms.gov/newsroom/fact-sheets/medicare-telemedicine-health-care-provider-fact-sheet.

Telehealth Resources for Patients and Clinicians From UCSF Center for Vulnerable Populations:

https://cvp.ucsf.edu/telehealth#

These include:

1. How to help patients download apps, set up Zoom meetings
2. Setting up a Zoom account for clinicians
3. Guide to your first telehealth visit
4. Sample clinical workflows
5. Reimbursement for Medicare and Medicaid

INDEX

N

O

P

Q

R

S

T

www.ingramcontent.com/pod-product-compliance
Lightning Source LLC
LaVergne TN
LVHW020934180325
806141LV00012B/463
* 9 7 8 1 7 9 3 5 4 9 9 4 5 *